Sutton,

I am thankful you are
in my class this year!
I hope you enjoy reading
my book! ♡,
        Mrs. Wenesday

Geeyahn What?

My Guillain-Barre' Syndrome Survival Story

Wenesday Ketron

Dedication

This book is dedicated to my amazing hubby, Greg; our awesome children, Ryan, Kayla, Sarah Grace, Kona, and Cindy; my fabulous mom and dad; all of my caretakers; my army of friends; GBS survivors around the world; and my sweet friend, Finis, who demonstrated his superhero strength and bravery by overcoming another rare autoimmune disease at age five during the time I was completing the final editing of my book.

Acknowledgements

Many thanks to Betsy, Shannon, Tonya, Sharyn, and Katy for helping with the tedious editing process and graciously listening to me talk about my book a lot.

A special thank you goes to the very talented David Humes, graphic designer extraordinaire, who designed my book cover. I gave him a picture that I had taken in Arizona of a winding road surrounded by rugged terrain. It was rough, with sharp rocks and pointy cactuses, but beautiful. I thought it was a great visual representation of my journey through Guillain-Barre' Syndrome.

The turtle has been adopted as an unofficial symbol for the GBS community. GBS is an acronym for Guillain-Barre' Syndrome and also for Getting Better Slowly. The turtle illustrates the slow, but steady and determined recovery. I asked David to combine the road and the turtle for my book cover. His vision far exceeded my expectations. I love the turtle intertwined with the road, determinedly trudging through the sand to survive, finding its way along its journey with a compass in the background.

Foreword

I had never before been so filled with fear, pain, and sadness; and later, joy and overwhelming gratitude. I want to share my story in order to provide others going through the journey of Guillain-Barre' Syndrome or any other life changing illness or event with hope, knowledge that they are not alone, and the promise of sunshine after the rain; caretakers with deeper understanding; and everyone with compassion for the fighters.

I wish to increase awareness of GBS. If even one person is diagnosed sooner because they or a family member recognized the early symptoms after reading this book and the progression of their syndrome is halted earlier rather than later; if someone finds hope in the depths of fear and despair; or if compassion is grown; my testimony will have served a worthy purpose.

Chapter 1

The End of My Denial

Carrie Underwood was standing in a pickup truck suspended by wires, moving over the crowd and over my head, singing beautifully. People all around me were singing along, smiling, and standing on their feet. I was enjoying the experience, her singing, the setting, but I was sitting down. I was weak and getting scared. Something was very wrong with me.

I was a thirty eight year old, healthy, full-time mom, attending the concert with my twelve year old daughter, Kayla, and my husband, Greg, at the Fed Ex Forum in Memphis, TN. I had looked forward to accompanying Kayla to her first concert since giving her the tickets months earlier on her birthday. I knew that if I couldn't shake off the feeling of malaise in this venue, I wouldn't be able to do so anywhere. Despite the excitement, I still felt something was very wrong physically, so I communicated this to Greg. We decided to leave a few minutes before the concert ended, trying to beat the mass exodus.

The stairs leading to the exit had never before looked so formidable. I held on tightly to the railing, determinedly, but clumsily swinging each leg up each step. It was very slow going. I glanced at the line that was forming behind me, worried that people would think I was drunk. All I saw was patience and concern on their faces. It was obvious to everyone else that something was physically wrong with me.

In the car, on the way home, I took a deep breath and told Greg, "I want to go to the emergency room tomorrow morning if I'm not any better." My legs were weak, I couldn't walk normally, my back ached, my extremities were numb and tingly, I was having difficulty going to the bathroom, my mouth tasted like a dirty copper penny, and I was uncomfortable. Greg was visibly relieved at my decision, wanting to get answers to what was happening to his wife. He answered, calmly, "Good. I think that's the right decision."

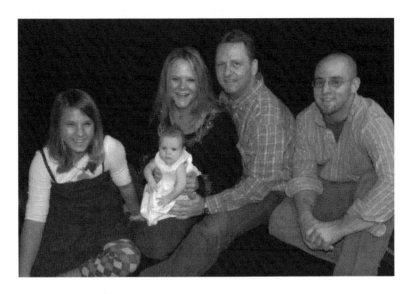

This family picture was taken about a year before I got sick. I always loved this photograph and my smile in it, well before I knew my smile was destined to change.

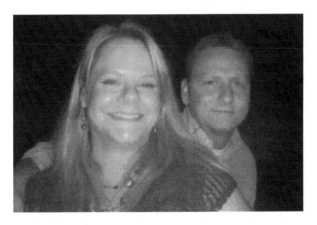

This picture was taken at the Carrie Underwood concert the night before I was hospitalized and paralyzed. This is the last picture I have of my original smile; my face was paralyzed the next day.

Chapter 2

In The Beginning and On the Bright Side

Prior to the concert, I'd had a stomach bug keeping me close to the bathroom for eight days. Diarrhea had never before been something that would cause me to visit the doctor; I rarely go to the doctor; but I had never had diarrhea last that long. On the eighth day, a Monday, I started vomiting too, so I visited my internist. He knew it was rare for me to go to the doctor, and he prescribed medication to stop the stomach symptoms and an antibiotic, Cipro, in case I had a bacterial infection.

Tuesday morning, when I woke up, my right big toe was numb and tingling, like it was asleep. It was odd because it didn't ever wake up over the course of the day. I mentioned it to my husband, but we both shrugged it off, not thinking an asleep big toe was any cause for concern.

By Wednesday, the tingling had spread into all ten toes and both feet, and my hands and tongue had joined in the act. I also had a yucky, metallic taste in my mouth that no amount of brushing, eating, or drinking would take away. I called my good friend, Jennifer, who was a nurse, and she thought I was probably having an allergic reaction to the Cipro, so I discontinued it.

On Thursday, none of my symptoms had subsided and my walking was beginning to look and feel odd. I didn't know how to describe it. I didn't know at the time that it was weakness in my legs. I could only label it as "weird." My walking was clumsy and uncoordinated; I couldn't walk in a straight line, and the stairs in my house were only possible to navigate if I held onto the railing. I have never been a person to think the sky is falling. In my experience, when I felt bad, I would start to feel better quickly. I didn't run to the doctor at the first sign of a sickness. This was enough though for me to know I needed to be evaluated.

My internist had no appointments available, so I visited an urgent care walk in clinic, where I was seen by a nurse practitioner I had never met before. She agreed that I was probably having an allergic reaction to Cipro. She gave me a huge steroid shot, sent me home with oral steroids, various allergy drugs, and a mouthwash for the weird taste.

By Friday, my walking had worsened – my mom described it as looking like I was a marionette. My hands, feet, and tongue were still numb, I still had that awful taste in my mouth, my back and neck started to feel stiff, and I'd started experiencing difficulty emptying my bladder. I left a phone message for my internist.

I carried my beautiful fifteen month old daughter, Sarah Grace, downstairs. A third of the way down, I collapsed. I didn't fall forward; my knees crumpled down onto the step on which I was standing. Somehow, I managed to hold on to Sarah Grace the whole time. She looked a little startled, but was unharmed. I stood back up, carefully finished walking downstairs with one hand on the railing, put my phone in my pocket for safety, and decided to stay downstairs for the rest of the day. Sarah Grace and I were home alone.

My internist returned my call that afternoon and I relayed all that had transpired since I last saw him. He was concerned and said that it didn't sound like an allergic reaction to him. He suggested I go to the emergency room. "Kayla's first concert of her life is tonight. We've been looking forward to it for months. Can I wait and see how I feel tomorrow and go to the emergency room if I'm not better?" I asked. My internist is usually jovial and laughing. His tone was more serious during this conversation. He responded, "If you go to the concert, just be sure to go to the emergency room if you start to get worse. If you don't start to improve, go to the emergency room tomorrow. I'm not sure what's going on without seeing you, but it does not sound like an allergic reaction to me."

I had looked forward to taking my daughter to the concert for so long, and we were so close, so I decided to go. When I told Greg what my doctor had said, Greg, my protector, wanted to take me the hospital immediately. "Kayla has looked forward to her first concert for five months. It's finally here. I just saw a doctor a couple days ago, who sent me home. I am fine. The ER will still be here tomorrow if I need it; Carrie Underwood won't wait for us," I said. Greg, knowing how stubborn I can be when it comes to finding a way to allow my children do something fun, responded, "I'll take Kayla and Tricia (Kayla's friend) to the concert while you stay home." I countered, "What difference does it make if I sit at home and feel bad or if I sit at the concert and feel bad? Either way, I'll be sitting, feeling bad, so I may as well do it while experiencing Kayla's first concert with her. This is something she will remember for the rest of her life." I had no idea how foretelling of a comment that was.

We live in Jackson, TN, and my parents live in Cordova, TN, about an hour away. It had been a huge blessing when they had been able to follow us to Tennessee from Louisiana only a year after we made that move. My mom was at our house to babysit Sarah Grace while we went to the concert. She was in Camp Greg, wanting me to stay home, but also understood my desire to go with Kayla. My dad, usually worry free, called me, "Wen, if you're feeling that crummy, you should really stay home." I explained to him too that it would make no difference if I felt crummy at home or at the concert, so I may as well experience the concert. I added, "The concert will be a welcome distraction from my feeling crummy, anyway. I'll probably even feel better if I go."

I am the epitome of an optimist. My experience in life has been that life is very good! Every time a storm comes, a rainbow brighter than ever imagined follows. I don't worry much. I am usually genuinely happy, content, and grateful. I've often thought if I could bottle whatever natural chemical surges through my body giving me peace and happiness, I'd sell it to the pharmaceutical industry and become a billionaire. I also love to have fun. Sometimes, Greg, who's more practical and doesn't always appreciate my sunny optimism leading to my bitter denial of potential consequences, calls FUN my "F-word." I'll forego cleaning the kitchen to go to the park with my kids in a heartbeat. I love playing and giggling, and I value quality time with my family above just about anything else.

7

There are pros and cons to my personality. My home is known as one with laughter, play dates, balloons, and messy cupcakes; but also dog hair, dirty dishes, and toy clutter. One of my favorite quotes is from the mom in the movie "Yours, Mine, and Ours" – "A home is for free expression, not good impressions."

On the plus side of my optimism, a couple years earlier, I convinced my best friend, Tara, and her husband, Josh, who live in Charlotte, NC, to load the car with our kids and drive thirty minutes to the Renaissance Festival when we were visiting, even though they objected because there was an eighty percent chance of rain and it was sprinkling a little. I said, "There's a twenty percent chance of sunshine! Twenty percent is quite good, really. If you had a twenty percent chance to win the lottery, you'd be ecstatic! If it rains a little, we won't melt; and if it pours, we'll leave. We should try!" The sky cleared just as we were parking, and we had a fantastic day of fun including jousting and magic shows. Tara and Josh started by complaining about my insistence, but went along, and ended up thanking me at the end of the day for dragging them out. We all had a blast.

On the flip side, several years ago, when my Uncle Howard called to say that I should go visit my grandma if I wanted to see her before she died, the downside of my optimism reared its ugly head. When I talked to Grandma Rose on the phone and asked her how she was feeling, her ninety two year old voice said, "Not too bad for a spring chicken." I knew in my heart she would be fine and my uncle was overreacting. She had always bounced back from every ailment in the past. Not flying to California the next day to visit her is one of my biggest regrets in life because she went to Heaven a few days later.

I insisted, so we decided that we would go to the Carrie Underwood concert as originally planned. Greg, Kayla, Tricia, and I playfully wrote Carrie's name on our car windows with window markers and started off on the hour and a half journey to Memphis with smiles on our faces. I explained to Tricia that I was having an allergic reaction to medicine and to not worry about me not being completely myself or walking totally normally. She said she understood, and she maintained a poker face, but her mother told me much later, "Tricia was really worried about you that night."

We took pictures at the concert. I had no way to know then that those photographs would be the last ever taken of my original smile. When they were taken, I thought, "Uh-oh, I am looking a little chubby. I should go on a diet," but I knew the pictures were important to remember Kayla's first concert and who was with her. Now, when I look at the pictures, all I see is all of our beautiful smiles. My top teeth are visible and both sides of my face look symmetrical. I don't see chubby now, I see beautiful. Life's surprises bring unexpected perspective.

Chapter 3

The Diagnosis

By Saturday morning, the day after the Carrie Underwood concert, it was clear that something was very wrong. Greg dropped me off at the emergency room door and parked the car. An ER worker saw my unusual gait and offered me a wheelchair, which I declined. Yes, my walking looked strange, but I thought to myself, "Certainly I don't need a wheelchair." Greg joined me in the waiting room, and we were immediately seen by a triage nurse. I'd heard horror stories of long ER waits, and expected to sit in the waiting room for hours.

I remembered waiting in the ER a few years earlier with Kayla – the only other time I'd ever been there. In our front yard, Kayla had handed her best friend, Ellie, her golf club. Ellie had been so excited to take a turn hitting the golf ball; she swung the club immediately, without thinking to wait for Kayla to clear the area. The club hit Kayla in the forehead, and she fell on the ground, her white shirt quickly turning red from all of the blood. Kayla cried in pain and Ellie cried just as much, feeling awful that her best friend was hurt. Greg and I drove to the ER without much concern for the speed limit. Kayla received her first – and last to this day – stitches. That wait with Kayla had seemed like an eternity.

This time, Greg drove me to the hospital without speeding. Ironically, my wait was shorter than Kayla's had been, only about fifteen minutes. I had apparently been triaged to fairly high on the priority list. My husband made productive use of our fifteen minutes and began searching my symptoms online from his phone. He came up with a diagnosis. He told me he thought I had Guillain-Barre' Syndrome. He even pronounced it correctly for me, using the pronunciation key he'd found – "Gee Yahn Bar Ray."

According to the National Institute of Neurological Disorders and Stroke, *"Guillain-Barré syndrome (GBS) is a disorder in which the body's immune system attacks part of the peripheral nervous system. Symptoms can increase in intensity until certain muscles cannot be used at all and, when severe, the person is almost totally paralyzed. In these cases the disorder is life threatening - potentially interfering with breathing and, at times, with blood pressure or heart rate - and is considered a medical emergency. Such an individual is often put on a ventilator to assist with breathing and is watched closely for problems such as an abnormal heart beat, infections, blood clots, and high or low blood pressure. Guillain-Barré syndrome can affect anybody. It can strike at any age and both sexes are equally prone to the disorder. The syndrome is rare, however, afflicting only about one person in 100,000."*

I love Greg with all of my heart. He and I have always said we're yin and yang. We're opposites, but together, we perfectly complete each other. Greg takes life seriously. I joke around a lot. Greg's ready to respond at a moment's notice. I have been told many times that I'm the most laid back person people have ever met. Normally, my reaction would be to say that I didn't have some exotic disease that we'd never heard of and that most people couldn't pronounce; I'd call him a worrier. That thought automatically surfaced, but only for a fraction of a second, and it was gone before I could even give voice to it. This time, I thought he might be right. I had a dread, despite trying to put it out of my head, that whatever was wrong with me was serious. This time, when the wheelchair was offered, I allowed myself to be pushed in it to the exam room.

The nurse quickly determined that I was dehydrated, so I was lying on the exam table with IV fluids entering my arm when the ER physician first laid eyes on me. Greg and I told the doctor everything that had been happening. Greg added, "I think my wife has Guillain-Barre' Syndrome." The doctor responded, "GBS is extremely rare. I doubt that's what's going on, but we will check it out."

The ER doctor checked my reflexes. I sat on the side of the bed while the doctor tapped my knees with a hammer-like tool. My legs didn't flinch at all. He seemed intrigued, and ordered a nerve conduction study.

I'd heard of nerve conduction studies, and I'd heard they were painful. The tech explained that essentially, she was going to place two electrodes on me, shock me, and determine how long it took for the signal to travel through my nerves from one electrode to another. It hurt a little, but I was relieved that it didn't hurt as much as I'd expected. I didn't know enough to be worried when it didn't hurt that much. She did the procedure in several places on my feet and legs. I asked her what the test told her, and she answered that the doctor would have to be the one to discuss the results with me. Ever the optimist, I questioned, "but it is normal, right?" She looked at me kindly and empathetically, and gently said, "No." My heart sank. A feeling of dread was starting to envelope me. Something really was wrong.

The ER doctor returned to deliver his news: based on what he knew thus far, he thought I did indeed have Guillain-Barre' Syndrome. On October 23, 2010, I was officially admitted into Jackson Madison County General Hospital with a diagnosis of GBS. The ER doctor ordered some other tests – a spinal tap and an MRI – to get confirmation and to rule out other (even worse) possibilities. The emergency physician asked Greg if he'd had any medical training, which he had not, and he shook Greg's hand. Apparently, my husband had become the talk of the ER because a few different doctors and nurses came into the ER exam room where I lay on the bed and said that they wanted to meet the husband who diagnosed his wife's Guillain Barre' Syndrome.

Greg had a little grin on his face. I had to join in his smile. It was pretty cool that my layman husband, in fifteen minutes, armed only with a cell phone, diagnosed what the medical professionals had not. For just a little while, we allowed ourselves to bask in the moment - Greg was a medical prodigy – or a cell phone research genius - and not to worry about what the diagnosis might actually mean.

A spinal tap sounded scary. I'd seen them done in various medical dramas on TV, and the person getting them always looked like he or she was in pain. It was explained that a needle would be inserted between two vertebrae and some cerebrospinal fluid would be removed. Once the doctor positioned me, I was told not to move. The doctor didn't have to tell me that twice. I didn't want to end up paralyzed. Nobody had said that could happen, but a needle was being placed in my spine!

I was nervous, but surprisingly, it was less painful than anticipated. The first shot stung for only a second – like a bee sting. Then, I felt a sheet on my back, and I felt pressure, but not really pain. The doctor told me exactly what he was doing as he did it, which was reassuring. I couldn't help but worry though that if I moved wrong, something bad would happen. So, I stayed still, and as a stereotypical coping mechanism, I found my happy place. I closed my eyes and drifted off to Saint Thomas. That's where Greg and I had gotten married four and a half years earlier. The water was clear and blue, the temperature was perfect, and love was in the air. We were surrounded by family and friends. There were no worries; there was only peace. The distraction worked, and the procedure ended. I was later told that my spinal fluid had contained excess protein, a hallmark of Guillain-Barre' Syndrome.

I was treated to my first MRI. I'd never had one before and had wondered what all the fuss was about. I'd heard of people complaining that MRIs sparked claustrophobia, and I'd seen new open MRI machines advertised. This machine was apparently not an open type. I was given an injection of dye to make the pictures from the test clearer. While my legs were out in the open air, my head was enclosed in a tunnel. I was again told to remain very still. This time, there was no fear that movement would cause injury, but that movement would cause the pictures to be blurry and the entire, long (about forty five minutes), process to be repeated. I remained as still as humanly possible.

The technician was in another room because of the radiation and talked to me through a microphone. The machine was incredibly loud, despite the earplugs. I heard repetitive tapping, thumping, and other strange noises. During one cycle, the machine seemed to yell in a deep voice, "Die! Die! Die! Die! Die!" The foreboding was increasing. I tried to interpret the sound differently, to hear it as saying something else, but that cycle clearly said, "Die!" and nothing else. The other cycles were just meaningless sounds.

I transported myself again to St. Thomas. Greg and I rode in a kayak in that gorgeous blue water. He did the paddling, and I just sat there, feeling the warmth of the sun and the protection of my husband sitting in front of me, driving the boat. I could look back toward the beach and see Kayla safely and happily playing in the sand with Grandma and Grandpa. Greg and I splashed water on each other and laughed. We joked about climbing aboard a yacht that was anchored nearby in the middle of the open water. The MRI finally ended.

The ER doctor told us that my GBS diagnosis was confirmed, and that my care would be transferred to an excellent neurologist. We were then introduced to Dr. Misulis, who had a friendly bedside manner and a big smile. After saying hello to me, Dr. Misulis shook Greg's hand and said, "so, you're the guy who diagnosed Guillain Barre'!" Yes, my husband was a legend!

Dr. Misulis talked to Greg and me while I was being wheeled to a private room. He told us that in addition to being a neurologist, he was in a band, which made him seem less like a distant physician and more like a real person. He gave us an overview of Guillain-Barre' Syndrome and what we might expect. While the medical information was provided in terms that we could understand, it was a lot to digest, and it was clear that this was not something to be taken lightly.

I called two of my good friends, Jennifer and Holly, who worked in that hospital and my cousin, Rob (who I think of as my brother), who is the head of the ER in his Massachusetts hospital. I wanted to be sure I could trust this doctor and I wanted him to know that I had medical professionals in my corner. I'm not usually a name dropper, but this felt like a great time to become one. My cousin, Rob, offered to speak to Dr. Misulis. Calling a patient's cousin thousands of miles away was a little above and beyond, and Dr. Misulis did it immediately. As silly as it sounds, that simple gesture signaled to me that I could trust this doctor and that things were going to be OK. After their phone call, Rob called me with reassurance, "Dr. Misulis sounds like he's very competent and knowledgeable about GBS. I believe you're in good hands. Call me if there's any medical jargon you need translated or if you have any concerns. I hope you start to improve soon!"

Chapter 4

Paralysis

Later that day, a lunch tray was placed in front of me in my private room. The roll looked good – it was one of those big, fluffy, fattening, normally very yummy and indulgent, white rolls. I hadn't eaten or drunk much at all in a few days because of the awful metallic taste in my mouth. I knew I needed sustenance, so I had kept trying. I took a bite of the roll. It felt like cotton in my mouth, but with a metallic taste. That taste made everything – even water – truly disgusting. I chewed on that piece of bread and tried to swallow it, but it just broke into pieces in my mouth. I had a mouth full of tiny pieces of cotton that tasted like metal. I couldn't swallow it. I spat it into a napkin.

I had to go to the bathroom. My mom had come to the hospital with my daughters, and they were in my room too. The nurse had shown me a potty seat by the bed. There was a bathroom in my room though, only a couple feet from my bed. Of course, I insisted on going to the real one. I held tightly onto Greg's arm, and once I was seated, he left the room. I hadn't been able to fully empty my bladder in a couple of days, and this time was no exception. As I stood up, my legs gave out and I collapsed onto the floor with a loud thump. My foot hit the hard porcelain toilet base as I fell. Then, I couldn't move my legs! I couldn't move my legs at all! And my foot hurt where it had hit. I screamed in my head, "Oh, my God! Help me!"

Before I could get any words out of my mouth, almost instantly, Greg was right there. He'd heard my fall. My mom had too, and she was screaming loudly for the nurse. Greg looked at me compassionately and told me he was going to pick me up off the floor. Terrified and wide-eyed, I said, "I can't move my legs! I can't help you! I can't support any of my weight! I don't know if you can pick me up." So far, Greg had been helping me walk, but I'd been helping too. Now, I couldn't move my legs. He quietly said, "I know. It's ok. I've got it. I promise I can pick you up." As he was lifting me, the nurse appeared. The two of them got me back into the bed. I couldn't move my legs. I couldn't move my legs. I couldn't move my legs or even my toes! The nurse said it was just a part of Guillain-Barre'. This was my first taste of the real, serious, effects of GBS. I was stunned. They'd said this could happen, but I didn't really expect it. I didn't like it. I hated it. It was awful!

Greg slept in my hospital room that night. My mom stayed at our house with Kayla and Sarah Grace. My mom and dad took turns visiting me with and without the girls. In that room, there were no visiting restrictions. Greg remained by my side. I don't know if it was because of the loss of my regular routine, the shock of all that was transpiring, the fear, the medicine, or the disease process, but the passage of time started to get fuzzy for me. It's unsettling lying there, just waiting to see if I would get worse, and just how bad I would get, with nothing that I could do to help myself and stop any progression.

At some point during the next day, Greg noticed that half of my face had fallen flat. He was clearly studying my face, and when I asked why he was staring at me, he said, "one side of your face isn't moving." I was confused, "What do you mean? My face doesn't feel any different." He called the nurse, and she agreed with him. One side of my face had become paralyzed – without my even being aware of it. I didn't know what to think – that was just weird – but, I did know it wasn't good. Later that day or the next, Greg and the nurse noticed that the other side of my face had fallen too.

I had gone from walking (albeit with assistance) and smiling (and taking that for granted) to not being able to move my legs or toes, not being able to sit up, and having my entire face paralyzed, all in a very short time, less than twenty four hours. Dr. Misulis visited and explained that while quite rare, bilateral facial paralysis can be caused from GBS, and that it is usually only temporary. "I don't know for sure, but I anticipate that your face will be back to normal once the GBS has run its course."

Unbeknownst to me, a call had gone out to let other people know about what was happening to me. Greg had called the people closest to us, and they had called mutual friends, who had called their friends, and offers of help immediately began pouring in to my family. On Monday morning, I received two beautiful flower arrangements delivered to my hospital room. One of the flower arrangements was traditional and gorgeous. The other included a giant decorative spider perched upon the flower basket. I knew the hospital staff would think it odd, but it served its purpose and made me laugh. Gina, one of my more conservative friends, knew that Halloween was one of my favorite holidays. Even as an adult, I have always loved having an excuse to play dress up. A Halloween themed arrangement was appropriate at that time of year, and it did my heart good to know that Gina had chosen it for me. Greg told me that a third flower arrangement, from Jennifer, had been delivered to our house, and he would bring it to me.

Later that morning, I heard the nurse say something to Greg about me starting to decline more rapidly. I was suddenly terrified. This was not good. The perpetual optimist was feeling anything but optimistic. What else could go wrong? I started to cry as I was moved, still in the bed, to the Neurological Intensive Care Unit (NICU). Without any of my flowers.

Chapter 5

Welcome To the NICU

In the NICU, I was warmly welcomed by a team of friendly, confident nurses. There were only seven or eight rooms in the NICU. I felt like I was in capable hands under their care. Still, it was extremely scary. I was attached to a myriad of wires and tubes. Not being able to empty my bladder had been part of the gradual escalation of my GBS, so a catheter was placed. It seemed like the phlebotomists wanted to continually take more blood than could possibly be circulating in my body and it didn't take long for my veins to collapse. It was decided that a central line would be placed as soon as possible. I wore a heart monitor, an oxygen monitor, and had an IV providing me with IVIG (intravenous immunoglobulin) medicine and some nourishment. It was explained that the IVIG would replace the specific parts of my blood cells that were attacking my nerves with those specific parts from other people's blood, that wouldn't attack my body. Each IVIG treatment, I was told, was extremely expensive because it takes about ten thousand plasma donors in order to make each treatment. I needed five treatments. I was grateful to fifty thousand donors.

My heart rate was erratic, especially while I was asleep, which alarmed the nurses, dropping sometimes into the low twenties. The potential need for a temporary pace maker was discussed, and I was introduced to my cardiologist. Dr. Cherry proved to be a very caring physician, who was clearly genuinely concerned about how I was doing both physically and emotionally. I told him,

"I'm scared, unable to move most of my body, hurting some, and becoming fuzzy about what time or day it is. I really need to get home soon. I have two children who need me at home. I'm a full time mom." He explained, "I wish we could do something more proactive. With GBS, we have to let it run its course and keep you as stable and comfortable as possible. The IVIG Dr. Misulis started for you should stop the progression sooner than what would be the case without that medicine. I wish I could offer more. I know it's frustrating for you." He explained what all would be involved with a temporary pace maker should it become necessary. "I hope it doesn't become necessary, but I'm here and we have a plan in case it does."

It was feared that my breathing muscles could become paralyzed, and that I might need to be put on a ventilator to breathe, so I was introduced to my pulmonologist (who turned out to be a mom from Kayla's school). Dr. Hagar went out of her way to make sure I was as comfortable – or at least in as little discomfort – as possible. She explained to me what would happen should the need for a ventilator arise. She said that she would constantly monitor my breathing capacity.

I was told that the sooner my legs were moved for me – even passively – and the sooner I exercised my arms, the better I would be in the long run. I was introduced to my physical therapist. Liz ended up being one of my favorite care takers during my entire ordeal – knowledgeable, compassionate, and creative, willing and eager to go the extra mile for me. Liz looked tall, but I had never stood next to her. She was younger than me, thin, had short brown hair, and was full of energy and enthusiasm.

While my neurologist was the doctor in charge of my care, there were a lot of professionals caring for me, and someone had to keep them all communicating with each other; therefore, I was introduced to my hospitalist. Dr. Lofton always wore a warm smile.

The nurses told me that I had the best room in the place. I was given the largest room, the one that was reserved for patients who were expected to have the longest stays. Greg brought pictures from home, and I was able to turn my head to the right and see my girls and my husband smiling at me from behind glass. The nurses hung cards I'd been receiving on the window blinds; there was a window in front of me with a view of the nurses' station. There was a window to the outside world to my left, with a nice view of distant trees. On my first day, the trees were still green.

I was terrified, unable to move my legs or toes, with no trunk control, unable to sit, uncomfortable, and exhausted. My arms and hands had begun to weaken, and it was feared that they could become as paralyzed as my legs. The nurse wiped my tears. I had not even been aware of the fact that I'd been crying. Apparently, I hadn't stopped crying since being moved into the NICU.

Everything was foggy. I was in disbelief that this was happening. I was a healthy thirty eight year old with no previous medical issues of any kind. I had just completed a series of boxing boot camp exercise classes. I had only stopped nursing my beautiful baby three months before getting sick. Nursing was supposed to be healthy for the baby AND mom. I had nursed for an entire year. My Sarah Grace should be in my arms and we should both be healthy. How could this be real? I was incredulous.

To top it all off, Greg was no longer permitted to stay with me around the clock. We would have to follow the visiting hours schedule in the NICU. This, I was told, was for my own good. Kayla and my parents could come only during visiting hours, but Sarah Grace was too young to visit at all. How could taking my most crucial support system away be for my own good? It would be good for me to have them all with me around the clock! This was a huge blow. I am very social and extroverted and love hugs. I don't typically covet alone time. I need my family and friends near me. I like to interact with other people.

I was getting weaker, and the discomfort in my body transitioned into real pain. My body was attacking my myelin, the outer covering of my nerves. I was told to expect things to get worse before they got better. That's how Guillain Barre' works. There's a fairly rapid decline, usually over the course of two to three weeks, followed by a plateau, and then a gradual recovery, which could be as fast as a few weeks or as long as a few years.

It was becoming obvious that I wasn't going home any time soon. I realized Greg would have to return to work. My mom had been staying at our house since I had been admitted to the hospital, helping Greg take care of our girls and our home. My mom worked, and I knew that she had my dad and their dog at home who would want her with them. My mom offered to retire early and move into our house for as long as needed.

I greatly appreciated her, and knew that we would accept the offer if needed, but I didn't want to think of the situation as long term. I didn't want my mom to give up her career to help me short term. I wanted a short term remedy, but I had no idea how to find it. I was a full time mom. Sarah Grace had never been in day care. We needed someone to care for Sarah Grace and play with her and to pick Kayla up from school and make sure she did her homework. It was impossible. My children needed me to be healthy and to be home!

I tried with every fiber in me, but I could not wiggle a single toe or move a leg muscle. I was given anti-anxiety medicine, anti-depression medicine, and pain medicine. It's rare for me even to take Ibuprofen or drink a glass of wine, and I am a vegetarian. Naturally, my stomach objected to all of the drugs, and I vomited. There wasn't much because I hadn't been eating, but since I couldn't sit up, it scared me. I didn't want to die from choking on my vomit as I lay flat in a hospital bed. My mouth was suctioned, like at a dentist's office. Things were starting to get truly miserable. I have a high threshold for discomfort, but there was a lot on my plate.

I could feel my body shutting down. It was getting difficult for me to fully open my eyes, even though they didn't fully close because of the facial paralysis. When the doctors tried to raise the back of the bed, in order to allow gravity to help my lungs function properly, it caused excruciating pain due to the damage to my nerves, so I lay totally flat in the hospital bed at all times.

People with GBS experience pain in a variety of ways. I now know that about eighty percent of GBS patients report pain to varying degrees. Some have such a severe reaction that even clothes or sheets touching their skin causes burning. In GBS, the body attacks and destroys the covering surrounding the nerves, and sometimes even the nerves themselves. The damage causes nerve signals from the brain to travel more slowly, to function irregularly, or to stop working all together. It is common for GBS patients to experience pain that is exacerbated with exercise. Movement of my body, even when powered by someone else or the back of a mechanical bed since I couldn't do it myself, was a form of exercise, and it produced a lot of pain.

I felt like I was dying. I asked the nurse, "Am I going to die?" He answered, "People can die from Guillain-Barre', but it is extremely rare, and I don't expect it to happen to you." That wasn't good enough. I wanted to hear that I definitely wasn't going to die.

I prayed – or more like pleaded, "Please, God, please let me get better! Please don't let me die! Please let me live to see my girls grow up and graduate from college and possibly graduate school or medical school. Please let me see them get married and have children. Please, God, my children need me! They need their mom! And I need to be with them! Please!" I was full of fear and desperation.

The nurse informed me that it was time to have my central line placed. A central line was something I had heard of in medical dramas on TV when patients were critically ill. I was told it would be placed in my neck and go into my heart, allowing medicines quick access to my blood stream and allowing the phlebotomists to bypass the collapsed veins in my arms. It would actually make things easier for me and for my body, which is why I had agreed to do it when it was recommended. I hadn't anticipated the anxiety I would have over the procedure. I had imagined Greg would be with me, holding my hand. I was told that I had to go immediately, that there was no time for Greg to be called and for him to drive to the hospital from work. He had known the procedure was going to happen – we had discussed it – we just hadn't known when.

Fortunately, my dear friend, Holly, who happened to be a surgical nurse in the hospital and was able to visit even when it was not official visiting hours, was in my room when the transport worker came for me. She went with me. She was a godsend who literally held my hand during the procedure.

I was terrified that something might go wrong, that after the central line was placed, I might lose use of my arms and hands and I might need to be placed on a ventilator, unable to talk. Fear gripped me. If I couldn't use my hands, I couldn't write; if I were on a ventilator, I couldn't speak. What if I couldn't communicate? What if I died? My tears were streaming and I could barely breathe. I was on the verge of a full blown panic attack, something I am not typically prone to having. Holly asked the person putting in the central line if I could have a piece of paper and a pen. I quickly scribbled notes to all three of my children – my one year old daughter, my twelve year old daughter, and my twenty five year old stepson – telling them that I loved them. Then, Holly squeezed my hand and kept me distracted while the central line was placed in my neck and down into my heart. The procedure was flawless. None of my fears materialized. I survived the central line placement. It didn't even hurt much physically, just emotionally. A flood of relief washed over me.

After Sarah Grace was born, she had stayed in the neonatal intensive care unit (NICU) for a little over a week because her blood sugar levels were not in the safe range. One morning, the nurses told me that they had tried to put a central line in her stomach, but that it coiled up in her liver, and they would probably have to put one in her neck in order to get the medication into her heart. I didn't know the anatomy, but I knew that I didn't want my precious baby to have to endure such a procedure. I had prayed then that God let me take her place – to make it so that she didn't have to have a central line, and to let me get it instead. I knew at the time my prayer didn't make a lot of sense, but it's what I prayed. Sarah Grace ended up not needing the central line at the last minute. A year later, I found myself in the neurological intensive care unit (NICU) with a central line, out of the blue. If I could have known for sure it was because I was taking Sarah Grace's place, I'd have embraced that central line and the whole ordeal with open arms and eagerness. As any parent, I would much rather feel pain and fear than have to witness my child go through it. I couldn't know if that was really what was happening, but it sort of made sense, and the idea was comforting to me.

The next event happened when I was by myself, some days later, after the risk of pneumonia had diminished. The nurse put a feeding tube in my nose, and as I gagged, down my throat. He apologized and a female nurse held my hand. There was no way to do it gently, so they did it quickly. I was given sore throat spray, which I ended up using every day the feeding tube was in; the tube irritated my throat, apparently a common side effect.

When Greg visited me, he made sure to confirm in my presence that no animals had been hurt in the making of my nourishment. It was vegetarian. I smiled internally because he'd thought to ask that for me.

Four different GBS survivors visited me at different times. I believe they heard about me from friends of friends, one of the benefits of living in a fairly small community. They each told me their stories of their diagnoses, treatments, and most importantly, recoveries. All but one were walking. One man was permanently in a wheelchair. None had facial paralysis, although none of them had at any point. Each offered understanding and hope. Each offered empathy like nobody else could and answers to many of my questions. One, an infectious diseases physician in the hospital, had the cruel recurring form of GBS and had gone through it multiple times. Even she was living, breathing, smiling, standing, walking, talking, and working. It was a blessing meeting these survivors.

They all said that they continued to have some variation of numbness or tingling in their toes. I can draw upon what they told me then, even now, several years later, to know that my continued numbness and tingling in my toes is normal with GBS and to not be afraid of it. They inspired me. Even while lying in the hospital bed fighting my GBS, I hoped that one day I could help others going through it, just as these angels had helped me.

Chapter 6

Monitors, Tubes, and Wires

I lay flat, staring at the wall to the right of my hospital bed, unable to move. To my left was a window and while I love the outdoors, between the window and me was the monitor, constantly beeping. It was filled with numbers, words, and graphs; and my finger and chest were attached to it with wires and cables. Often, it would beep loudly and urgently, signaling an emergency and any nurse who was with me would dart out of the room and head to the person who'd been identified on my monitor as having stopped breathing, and I'd be reminded again what a serious place I was in. My monitor displayed largely my vital statistics, but there was a corner reserved for a code to show up if any of my fellow NICU patients were in distress.

I hated that monitor. I didn't understand what everything on it meant, but I knew that it told of my oxygen levels that constantly needed to be watched and my heart rate, which dipped periodically too low for anyone's comfort. I also had a feeding tube in my nose, an IV in my arm, and a central line in my neck. Those tubes were attached on my right, and I don't know why or how, but it seemed if I looked to the left, everything would get tangled. So, I looked straight ahead or to the right, but avoided the left as much as I could, even though that was where the window was that led to the outside world, the real world, that I loved and missed. It was the window with the view of the green tree leaves turning orange and brown.

My world was suddenly contained in a tiny room. There were no children, no toys, no schedules of places I needed and wanted to be - just a bed, my painful body, wires, tubes, beeping on the monitor, and a TV that I couldn't focus on enough to even watch. I had no idea how much time had passed since I'd been admitted into the hospital. Time lost all meaning for me, and yet it seemed to drag by very slowly. It was depressing thinking of all the activity that was going on outside, activity I very much wanted to be a part of again, contrasted with the nothingness going on in my room.

With my facial paralysis came bug eyes. That wasn't a term I heard until much later, when people felt more comfortable joking with me, after the fact. My facial paralysis caused my eyes to remain wide open – and to remain partially open even while I slept. That caused my eyes to become acutely dry and my vision to become blurry. The ophthalmologist who visited reassured me that he expected the blurriness to only be temporary. The nurses offered to tape my eyelids shut while I slept, but that sounded like something from a horror movie, so I declined. Eye cream and eye drops were regularly placed in my eyes.

I was completely helpless, dependent on everyone else for everything. A cleaning lady came periodically to sanitize my room. She was perky and talkative, and didn't seem to mind that I couldn't smile back at her. Nevertheless, I apologized for not being able to smile. She asked me one day if I liked the newscaster's hairstyle on TV. I answered, "I do. I think it looks a lot like yours!" Her eyes lit up. I got the impression that was exactly what she'd hoped to hear. She looked at my pictures in my room, and then she asked, "Have you seen yourself since you've been in here?" I simply responded, "No." She offered me a mirror from her pocket.

The reflection I saw was not me. It was a pale, wide eyed lady with oily hair and an ugly tube going into her nose and bandages on her neck with tubes coming out of them. The lady in the reflection looked like she was on her death bed. It was awful. I decided not to look in a mirror again or have any pictures taken as long as I was in the NICU. I knew the mirror had been offered as a kind gesture, so I held my tears back until she left the room.

My voice was weak and very slurred from the paralysis. People had great difficulty understanding what I was saying. Those who know me know that such an impediment couldn't stop me from trying. My family, close friends who visited, nurses, and doctors made great efforts and were very good at focusing on what I was saying, sparing me from grasping the extent of my poor speech. My dad joked, "I can understand you better than ever because you are trying so hard to speak clearly and deliberately, and not jibber jabbering away, as usual."

One day, a team of nursing students entered my room with a teacher who was obviously excited about the opportunity to show them a patient with Guillain Barre Syndrome. I felt like I was in an episode of "Grey's Anatomy." I thought it would be more educational for the nursing students – and fun for me – if I told them my story, rather than have the teacher just read to them from my chart. All eyes and ears were on me. With detail and enthusiasm, I began my story. I was feeling pretty good being able to teach. Then, the teacher repeated, in questioning form, something she thought I had said. I'd said something to the effect of, "I fell down on the floor." She asked something like, "you called your husband on the phone?" She had not understood a word of what I had said. None of them had. That was really frustrating and really depressing. I closed my eyes and tried to drift off to sleep to escape.

Sleep was not easy. Phlebotomists had stopped taking blood from my veins, because they were able to get it from the central line, but the pulmonology technicians started waking me around the clock to test my lung capacity. I had to blow and suck into plastic tubes. The challenge was that with my facial paralysis, I wasn't able to form a seal with my lips around the tubes, so the results of those tests were flawed. It was a relief when I had the same tech more than once, but often, especially in the middle of the night, I would get someone new, and the nurses and I would have to explain again that I couldn't form a seal with my lips. Some of the technicians tried to get creative and invent a mouthpiece that would work using the materials they had. Others just seemed confused by it all.

They also took X-rays of my lungs. That required the techs raising the back of my bed, which in itself caused incredible pain in my back, shooting down into my legs. They then placed a metal board behind me while they left the room and pushed a button to take a picture. They were very compassionate and I could tell truly felt bad for causing me pain. They lowered the bed as quickly as possible immediately after pushing the button, but it was long enough to cause burning in my entire body. It hurt to be upright, even when it was not my muscles doing the work.

I was exhausted, but unable to close my eyes completely, and I couldn't seem to get a solid stretch of uninterrupted, pain free sleep. At the same time, I couldn't keep my eyes open and stay fully awake. It was a surreal paradox. I could feel my body shutting down, and I couldn't do anything about it.

I knew that despite all the efforts, there was a real possibility that I could die in that room. In the movies, a dying person's life flashes before her eyes in an instant. My life flashed before my eyes, but it did so over a period of days, not seconds.

Chapter 7

Memories

I was eight years old, halfway through third grade. My parents and I were standing just inside the tunnel that led from the terminal into the airplane. I hesitated, knowing I would miss my best friend, Tara, who was still waving from the terminal end of the jet way. My dad asked, "Don't you want to go?" I didn't want to hurt his feelings. I put on a brave smile, held his hand, and walked forward, toward the airplane that would take us across the Pacific Ocean to our new home in the Philippines.

I opened my eyes and saw Liz, my physical therapist, standing next to my bed, smiling. I wanted to work with her. I wanted to do it so that I could get stronger and get home to my family sooner, and I didn't want to disappoint Liz. I just couldn't keep my eyes open. I didn't have the strength. I asked if we could work with my eyes closed. She put her hand on my arm and said, "If it's ok with you, it's ok with me. I'm glad you're so motivated to get better that you're willing to work even with your eyes shut. This will help you." She moved my legs slowly up and down while I lay there with my eyes shut, drifting in and out of consciousness.

Being a kid in the Philippines was fun! I lived there from the middle of third grade through the end of sixth grade. Turning ten years old marked a huge milestone – it was when the children who lived on the base got their official identification cards. Having an ID opened a world of independence – with an ID, a kid could rent a go cart, ride a horse, shop alone at the Exchange (the main store on base), travel solo on base transportation, etc.

My best friend, Margo, and I loved mysteries. We would take a shuttle boat to Grande Island (a small island, part of the navy base, dedicated to recreation). There, we would rent bikes and set off on adventures. We'd spy on construction workers and groundskeepers and concoct all kinds of stories about them. One time, we convinced ourselves the workers we were watching were part of a murder mystery.

We peeked through the glass of a work shed a little off the bike path. When the workers spotted us, our hearts pounded, "They know we're out here!" We jumped on our bikes, and were in such a hurry to get out of the area, we actually crashed into each other and fell! We cracked up laughing, got back up, and pedaled as quickly as we could, with no real destination, and wound up in eyesight of an abandoned World War II hospital. Naturally, we ditched our bikes and ran toward it.

There was no electricity and it was a perfect place for our imagined murder mystery plot to unfold. There were even old, rusty bedframes still in some of the rooms. "This is where those guys take their victims to kill them!" We ran through that building with lightning speed, and jumped back on our bikes. We pedaled to a restaurant, where we discussed and wrote down everything we had seen over hamburgers and french fries (I was a meat eater then). "There were five men. They got jobs as gardeners here because that would give them the perfect cover to have their weapons out in the open. Did you see all the knives in the work shed? I think they had at least twenty. They had four or five machetes too!" At the end of the day, we boarded the shuttle boat and went back home.

When I was about eleven years old, still living in the Philippines, we participated in "family day" on an aircraft carrier, the USS Constellation, in the South China Sea. We stood outside, on the bridge, as the planes took off and landed in front of us. The heat was intense from the plane engines and we could feel it! They were loud too! A small battleship pulled up next to us and sailors demonstrated how they could climb on ropes from one vessel to the other. The ship had an entire room filled with video games, and in the days before computers, tablets, and cell phones, that was very cool.

The best part of that day was the demonstration of bombs being dropped. We were told to cover our ears. I held my hands over my ears, saw the flashes of light at the surface of the ocean, decided it wasn't really loud at all, took my hands down, and THEN heard VERY loudly, "BOOM! BOOM! BOOM!" It was a real life lesson that I remember clearly to this day – light travels faster than sound!

I also learned something about negotiating in the Philippines. Shopping off base meant negotiating at outdoor markets. There, full price was never paid for items. The method of shopping was called bargaining. We all had unique ways of bargaining, and we made a game of it to see who could get the best deal. My mom would ask how much something cost. When told ten pesos, she would ask if she could have it for eight. The vendor would counter with nine, and an agreement would be reached. If my dad were told something cost ten pesos, he would ask if he could have it for five. The vendor would say no, but that he could sell it for nine. My dad would simply walk away. Ninety percent of the time, the vendor would then chase after my dad and agree to sell the item for six pesos. Sometimes though, the vendor would get offended, not follow my dad, and no deal was struck.

I made use of my cute kid status. When I was told something cost ten pesos, I'd put on a pouty face and say, "I only have seven pesos." Usually, I'd get what I wanted at the price I asked. I went lower than my mom, but not as low as my dad. I usually bought unique erasers and pencil boxes to trade at school or figurines made out of shells to add to my collection.

My current adventure was not on a beautiful island and it was not fun. I tried negotiating in the hospital. I told God that if he made me better, I'd be a better person. I told Him that if he made me better, I'd help other people. I told Him that if he made me better, I'd be a better mother and wife. I told Him that if He made me better, I'd keep my home cleaner. I told Him that if He made me better, I'd go to church more regularly. I told Him I would do anything He wanted if He made me better.

After living in the Philippines for four years, we moved to Scotland the summer after sixth grade and lived there for three years, until the summer after ninth grade. Scotland was completely different from the Philippines. There were no barbed wires keeping us safely confined inside the boundaries of a base. Most people where I lived in Scotland didn't even lock their doors regularly. The Philippines had been home to monkeys living in the jungles surrounding our neighborhoods. In Scotland, there were fields filled with rabbits surrounding our neighborhoods, and sometimes I'd find a hedgehog on the side of the road. In the Philippines, it was always hot, and it rained only during rainy season; in Scotland, it was always cold and it constantly rained. Scotland was home to beautiful fields dotted with sheep, centuries-old castles, and the tastiest sweet shops I'd ever visited, where chocolate was bought by weight. In the Philippines, young men wore pants and barongs (dress shirts) to weddings; in Scotland, young men wore kilts to weddings and we kids occasionally stuck mirrors on our shoes to see what was under the kilt.

We lived in a wee Scottish village, Edzell, and then in a small Scottish city, Brechin. I went to a Scottish school (seventh through ninth grade, or as it was called there, first through third year). The only Americans I saw regularly were my parents. I quickly picked up a very strong Scottish accent. Even my Scottish friends forgot that I was American and any new Scottish people I met didn't know I was American. They were always shocked when they met my parents, who spoke with strong American accents.

I loved living in Scotland. I joined the other kids my age picking strawberries in the summers and potatoes in the winters. Kids provided cheap labor for the farmers and the farmers provided pocket money for the kids. I saved my earnings and bought my first ten speed bike. It was a red Kalkhoff (a German make). I was so proud of that bicycle because I had bought it with my own money. I kept it until I was thirty, even though by then, it had completely rusted.

I remembered looking out of the window in biology, watching the blizzard outside. The kids riding the Edzell bus were always among the first to be dismissed early because of the easily blocked country roads. We were excited, knowing the white outside meant that our bus would be called over the loud speaker. Mr. Baxter, our teacher, asked why we were all staring outside, and we excitedly exclaimed, "It's snowing hard! We're going home soon!" Mr. Baxter replied, "It's no!" In Scotland, saying, "it's no," is as grammatically acceptable as saying, "it's not." "Aye, it is," we answered. Then he laughed, "Aye, I said, 'it's snow!'" We all laughed at his play on words.

The snow blowing in the wind was cold and would sting our skin. Because we preteens were more concerned with fashion than warmth and comfort, we would wear heeled pumps on our feet instead of boots. Our feet would turn red, and then blue. Eventually, once inside a heated building, we would begin to thaw out. Our skin would burn and tingle. That's the feeling I experienced throughout my body in the hospital. My skin was burning and tingling, like it was thawing from having been frozen.

I am a touchy-feely person, who craves hand holding and cuddles from my loved ones. When my family visited me in the NICU, they'd hold my hand. The touch would intensify the burning and the tingling, but the emotional warmth made it worth it. It was a hurt that felt good. My nerves were damaged and sending mixed signals to my brain. Nothing my body felt made logical sense. Hugs were almost impossible since I was lying flat, attached to so many things, but hand holding was good for my soul.

I revisited my travels and life experiences in my mind, and spent a great deal of time thinking about my daughters. Their births marked the only times previously that I'd been hospitalized. Those hospitalizations had culminated in the births of my two favorite people in the world – Kayla and Sarah Grace.

Kayla was born when I was twenty six years old. She was the most beautiful thing I had ever seen in my life. The moment she popped out into the world, I announced, "She's perfect!" I had never before been so in love with another human being. I was thirty seven years old when Sarah Grace was born, and it was like I was having a baby for the first time again – equally perfect and equally majestic. Both of my girls had beautiful, soulful blue eyes (Kayla's later turned to a gorgeous deep green, and Sarah Grace's remained sea blue like her dad's), ten tiny fingers and ten tiny toes. Kayla had a headful of dark hair that subsequently fell out, and then grew back in very light blonde. Sarah Grace's hair was reddish blonde at first and later turned very blonde. Both were happy babies, full of love and peace and joy from the beginning.

My memories of their births and their young childhoods filled me with tears of joy. I enjoyed every minute of their lives – even the crying. All of the stages brought different novel experiences. All of the stages allowed their precious personalities to shine. I loved holding them. I loved watching them progress forward on their own. I loved making everything better with a simple kiss. I loved watching them laugh. I loved laughing with them. The jolting reality that I was not able to be with them filled me with tears of sadness.

I also thought very much about my relationship with my husband. We had both had life experiences, children, ex-spouses, and careers when we met. "Bless the Broken Road" by Rascal Flats is one of our theme songs. I am thankful daily that Greg's and my roads crossed and we met and fell in love.

Greg and I are opposites who attract. We are yin and yang. When we were dating, Greg took me on a cruise to Cozumel, where we swam with dolphins. Before we could get into the water, we had to watch an instructional/safety video. Greg watched intently, digesting every rule. I saw the people and dolphins on the screen and vaguely heard talking, but my internal voice was happily chirping, "Oh, my gosh! I cannot believe we are about to swim with dolphins! I have always wanted to swim with dolphins! This is going to be so cool! I love dolphins! I love Greg! We'll have to take pictures…."

Once in the water, the trainer asked for a volunteer to go first. My hand was in the air, and my feet were a foot off the ground, "Me! I'll go first!" I swam out to the point where the dolphin meeting was to take place. I knew there was something I needed to do, but what? I yelled, "Greg! What do I do?" He responded, "You should have paid attention to the video!" I answered, "Just tell me!" He shouted and provided animation, "Put your feet out like this, and put your arms out like this!" I did, and within seconds, I was being propelled through the water and into the air with two dolphin noses pushing against my two feet. It was majestic!

In the hospital, our personalities remained. I understood and could accept uncertainty. The doctors really didn't know how severe my Guillain-Barre' would get before I reached the plateau or when I would start to improve. I'm a go-with-the flow person, and that part of it made sense to me. We would have to take a wait and see approach.

Greg wanted concrete answers. Each time Dr. Misulis entered my room, Greg asked the same questions in multiple ways, trying to prompt the neurologist to provide answers. "Has she plateaued yet? When will she plateau? When do you anticipate she could plateau? How will we know when she plateaus? How bad will it get before she plateaus? Will she need to be on a ventilator? How will we know if she needs to be on a ventilator?" I could see Greg's frustration with not knowing. I could see Dr. Misulis' frustration with not having the answers to provide.

Chapter 8

One Answered Prayer

I was struggling with the theological implications of my suffering. I was constantly praying and pleading. "Please, God, please, keep me alive! My children need me. My husband needs me. Please let me get better. Please stop the pain. Please stop the burning. Please provide a solution to how to care for my children while I'm in the hospital. I'm not a saint, but I am a good person. I haven't done anything bad enough to warrant this."

One prayer was answered. Holly's husband (Holly had been with me when I had the central line placed), Steve, had a friend, Mike, whose girlfriend was taking a break from nursing school and looking for a nanny job. Greg had arranged for her to come to the hospital. Greg told me, "I think Stephanie's perfect! You are the final decision maker though as to whether or not we hire her. You are Kayla's and Sarah Grace's mom, and you have to love her for us to hire her. She's going to visit today so that you can meet her. I'll wait until she leaves, and then you can tell me what you think." I appreciated more than I could express that as helpless as I was, my husband blessed me with feeling like I had some control over what would happen with our children.

From the moment Stephanie walked into my room, I knew she was the one for the job. She was young and beautiful, and I knew instantly that her beauty was soul deep and not just skin deep. She had a genuine smile and made eye contact with me when we talked. She patiently focused on and understood what I said. She told me of her love for children of all ages, and I could feel the genuineness.

Of course I love my children, but I also love all children, in general. My favorite job I ever had wasn't the one I went through graduate school to do, but was the one I returned to every summer during high school and college. I had been a summer camp counselor and thoroughly loved it. I loved playing with and caring for children. I could tell instantly that Stephanie was a lot like me. She would keep my girls safe and happy. I knew Kayla and Sarah Grace would both love her. She was hired!

Stephanie was a gift from God dropped right into my hospital room. What was the likelihood that the timing would work out perfectly like it did, or that we would ever hear of her in the first place? And Greg told me that my parents had offered to help pay for our nanny. This time I prayed, "Thank you, God!"

As word was spreading that I was in the hospital, Greg's phone was ringing a lot. Offers from friends were pouring in to drive Kayla and Sarah Grace to their activities, to babysit, to help in any way we needed. Greg and I were humbled and very appreciative, but Greg was suddenly extra busy. Tara, my best friend since childhood, started a Caring Bridge website for us. Caring Bridge is an online presence where a host can offer updates about a sick person, and family and friends can leave notes for that person. This provided a convenient way for Greg to share information with everyone without being tied to the phone, and for me to receive many notes of encouragement. Each time Greg visited, during the official NICU visiting hours, he read to me the notes people had written.

I quickly began to look forward to hearing the messages – it felt really good to know that while not everyone could fit into the NICU during the short visiting hours, a whole lot of people cared about me and my family. Hearing from my people in this way became one of the things I looked forward to the most during Greg's visits. Some notes were very serious and some were light hearted. Some notes were from people I lived near, whom I normally saw on a regular basis; and some were from family thousands of miles away and friends I hadn't seen in years. Each one made me smile – internally.

The first note was from Tara. It simply said, *"I am sending you all the love and strength that I have to help you get through this!"* I was not alone.

A Take Them a Meal site was also started, where people signed up to deliver food to my family while I was in the hospital. I think my daughters, husband, and mom ate better during that time period than they did when I was at home. That also made me smile – internally.

Chapter 9

Visitors and Helpers

Time in the neuro ICU passed very slowly. I couldn't focus on the TV, and really wasn't interested in watching it. I looked forward to visiting hours more than anything else.

Shannon, my neighbor and closest friend in Tennessee, visited almost every day, often with her teenage kids, Eric and Ellie. Shannon always came in with a smile and news from my world. It was a couple years later when she told me that she used to return home or return to work crying after our visits. I was grateful for the smiles she showed me. Shannon brought me some dry shampoo (a spray intended to absorb oil), which made my head feel a little cleaner before that glorious day when my nurses washed my hair.

The dry shampoo was a lovely idea, and it helped, but I had washed my hair with running water, shampoo, and conditioner daily my entire life. I craved that squeaky clean feeling that I had taken for granted before. Since I was attached to such a myriad of medical equipment with wires and tubes, and sitting up was impossible for me on my own and excruciatingly painful with back support, how to wash my hair was a dilemma.

Two of my favorite female nurses, Leigh Ann and Jennifer, entered my room with big smiles. "We've talked about it, and have figured out a way to wash your hair! Everybody else in the ICU is doing pretty well right now, so we think we'll have time. If there's an emergency, we'll leave, but know we will return to finish your hair when we can." I nodded emphatically. They put towels and absorbent pads under my head, and poured water from a bowl over my tresses as I lay flat on the bed, smiling on the inside. They scrubbed my hair with shampoo and rinsed it, then added conditioner, and rinsed that out. They used a soapy washcloth to clean my entire body. They didn't get called away during the entire procedure. I was cold, but I was not complaining. I was clean! It felt great! They tucked me in with blankets when my bath was complete. Leigh Ann braided my hair in two braids on the sides of my head to prevent my hair from getting matted again. I imagined one day taking Leigh Ann and Jennifer to lunch to thank them.

Eugene and Randy, the head pastors at my church, visited. That was a first for me – having clergy visit in the hospital. I had mixed emotions of joy that they were there, and worry that they were there. I was happy and humbled that they loved me enough to visit – I was only one of thousands of members of our large church – and I was worried because I knew that it meant I was really sick. They asked how I was doing and didn't seem to mind that I didn't have the strength to keep my eyes open while talking to them. They held my hands and prayed with me. I wanted to ask them why this was happening to me, but I didn't.

I was starting to get angry with God for putting me through so much pain and for taking me away from my children. I wanted Eugene and Randy to tell me what the grand plan was, to let me know the reason for my suffering. I didn't have the strength to ask them though, and of course, I knew they couldn't have those answers.

Randy told me a story that will stick with me forever. I knew his son was in a wheelchair and had a significant disability, but I never knew exactly what it was and had never asked. Randy told me that when his son was very young, he was in the exact same neuro ICU room that I was in. Randy's son, Gordon, had been developing normally until he had a polio vaccine. He had a rare reaction to the vaccine and contracted polio. Randy said that at first, the doctors had thought Gordon had Guillain Barre' Syndrome, but then confirmed that it was in fact polio. Gordon's case was one of the reasons that the formulation used nationally in the polio vaccine was changed. I shed more tears – how awful that would have been to see his child in pain and not know why, and then learn that he would be forever disabled. I would much rather it be me suffering than my child or any child. It must have been emotional for Randy being in that same room again, talking to someone with GBS.

Our entire church was praying for me. One Sunday, while I was in the NICU, Greg visited me after church. He said that Randy had asked him to stand on the stage, and the whole congregation prayed for me and for Greg and for our children. We are not normally an on the stage in church couple. The outpouring of love and support that we received from our church family brought Greg and me both to tears – grateful tears.

Ray visited me almost every day. He was my friend's husband, an elder in our church, and a physician. The fact that he was a doctor meant that he was able to visit me during those moments when I was staring at the blurry clock, waiting for visiting hours to arrive. He held my hand and prayed with me, and talked with me, and made sure I was being well cared for. He'd ask the nurses and doctors for updates, and I found comfort knowing that he was looking out for me. It was much later that his wife confided in me that while Ray regularly visits a lot of our church members who are hospitalized; he had been truly worried about me. My condition had been grave.

Two friends from the Jackson Service League, our local equivalent of the southern Junior League, visited around Halloween. Ashley brought me a silver angel, which the nurse hung on my IV stand. Taylor, knowing how much I love to dress up at Halloween and insist that everyone else dress up too, visited wearing a costume wig. She made me laugh.

Then, one day, I was lying in bed, knowing that nobody was coming during that visiting hour. It was unusual and disappointing, but I understood. Life went on outside of the hospital for everyone else. I saw a group of teenagers walk past my window, into the room around the corner from mine. I believed from the visitors to that room that a teenager was the probable occupant. I often wondered what had happened to him or her, but never asked anybody, knowing they wouldn't be able to tell me because of confidentiality rules.

A large group of people crowded into the room across the hall from me. A rather large woman sang a gospel song, loudly and proudly. It was beautiful – a gift for everyone in earshot. Afterwards, the people in that room applauded. Those visitors didn't stay for long though. Shortly after the song, they each left the room one by one. I wondered about the patient in that room. It was the only other room in the NICU as large as mine, so I knew he or she was expected to be in there for a long time. I wondered if he or she had even been fully conscious while the woman sang. Either way, it was touching.

I saw a priest look right into my window. I knew he wasn't visiting me because I'm not Catholic. He walked into my room, and I opened my mouth to tell him he had the wrong room. Before I could get any words out, he cheerfully asked, "Are you Wenesday?" He did have the right room after all. He introduced himself and explained, "My name is Father Chuck. I'm Taylor's priest," (she belongs to an Anglican church) "and Taylor has been really concerned about you and asked me to visit." That Taylor cared so much, coupled with the obvious warmth in this man, warmed my heart. It was wonderful to know that my friend thought so much about me, and that this man was willing to drive to the hospital to see me and pray with me, even though I didn't know him or attend his church. The timing was perfect too – I ended up having a visitor when I had been feeling a bit lonely. And he returned more than once after that.

Heather is my beautiful friend, a full-time mom, former physical therapist. She visited one day, donning a pretty scarf, signaling to me that the season was changing outside and it was no longer the shorts weather it had been when I had arrived. She also came bearing a bag of practical gifts, including disposable toothbrushes and a notebook and pen. I first used the notebook and pen to ask my nurse to write the names of my care givers so that I could one day write them thank you notes, and later I used them to practice handwriting. I asked Heather to move my legs for me, knowing it would be beneficial. She completed the physical therapy routine of passive movement for me each time she visited. The more my limbs were moved, the better.

I was always thankful for my family and friends. Betsy was my college roommate and has been one of my closest friends ever since our days at Louisiana State University. As an art major, she used to try her hardest to get me to sit down and watch old movies with her, but I never had the patience. I like things to move a little faster than they did in the days before modern special effects. We used to joke about how Betsy enjoyed alone time, and I liked being in the thick of things around people. Betsy is a classic introvert, and I am definitely an extravert. We've always gotten along really well, sharing a common sense of humor. Betsy lives in Texas and has always known how to make me laugh. One of her Caring Bridge posts really made me feel good. She wrote, in part, *"You are NOT a girl who enjoys spending a lot of time alone...I know that's got to be one of the hardest parts of this. It kills me that I can't be there to visit, and you know I'd be bringing books and magazines and movies that I'd tell you that you would love, that you may or may not.... Ah, this would be one way to pin you down and make you watch 'Sense and Sensibility.' You've got to be massively frustrated and I hate it for you...you know everyone misses your eternal optimist flitting from flower to flower. Besides the fact that we got to catch up and had a lot of fun, I'm really glad I got to visit you in May, because now I can picture where you are, and some of the small army of friends who are helping you through this...."* Yes, she was right, I had a small army of family and friends, and they were indeed helping me through this. Having that fact pointed out made me very thankful.

Chapter 10

Facing the Grim Truth and Finding Peace

I could feel my body shutting down. I had not an ounce of energy. I could barely open my eyes and it was very difficult to focus and stay awake. My entire body hurt. I couldn't move most of my body, and my heart rate was very low. I knew deep down that I was dying. It was possible that my condition might start to get better, but I was keenly aware for the first time in my optimistic life that it truly might not.

I was beginning to have difficulty breathing, and the nurses put an oxygen mask on me. It wasn't the unobtrusive tube that sits beneath people's noses; rather, it was a bulky mask that covered my mouth and nose and was strapped tightly to my head. I was instantly claustrophobic and wanted it off. I didn't have the strength or dexterity to remove the strap myself, and the nurses refused to take it off of me without the consent of my pulmonologist. I was terrified that the next step would be a ventilator. That oxygen mask, rather than providing me with the intended comfort, worried and irritated me greatly.

I felt the overwhelming need to talk to Kayla. I had gotten Greg's blessing to have a serious conversation with my oldest daughter. Greg was there, holding Kayla's hand, while she and I talked. As I looked at my beautiful daughter, I said, "Kayla, I don't expect to die from GBS. It is possible though. Anything is possible. I want to tell you some things right now. I love you. I am so very proud of you. You are loving, smart, sweet, generous, kind, beautiful, funny, happy, and strong, and I want you to know that I truly love those things about you. I am thankful and proud that I have had the blessing of spending twelve wonderful years with you. You make me happy beyond words."

I also talked to Kayla about how grateful I was for Greg, and for Kayla's close relationship with her stepdad. Kayla was five years old when Greg and I began dating, seven when we got married. When Kayla was five, she used to steal Greg's hat each time he visited. She said, "I'll give it to you next time you come!" She'd confided in me, "That way, he'll have to come back!"

Greg has always been a stepdad to Kayla only on paper; he knows and respects that Kayla has a father, but in Greg's heart, Kayla is simply his daughter and not a distant "step." I told Kayla that if I were to die, it was extremely important to me for them to continue their relationship even after I was gone. They love each other and are mutually good for each other.

Of course, the same was true of Kayla and Sarah Grace. They are sisters with an eleven year age difference, but the closest two sisters I've ever seen. I also explained that every mother wants to teach her children about her views on life, that I was confident and joyful that Kayla understood and embraced mine, but that I was sad about the thought of possibly not being able to instill my essence in Sarah Grace. Greg loves me, but his yin does not always completely understand my yang. Kayla not only gets me, she is me to a certain extent – just a little shorter and a lot prettier.

I asked Kayla, "Please be sure, if I don't make it out of this hospital bed, to teach Sarah Grace about the world though my eyes, as only you can. Help her figure out what I might say or advise in a specific situation. I want Sarah Grace to learn to find true joy in life, be thankful for her blessings, experience a lot of laughter, know how to relax, have fun, prompt others around her to smile, value education, be a true friend, be trustworthy and honest, love wholeheartedly, be kind, try to understand both sides of an argument..." Kayla knew what I meant. I believed her completely when she agreed to instill those things in Sarah Grace and to constantly tell Sarah Grace that I loved her. I was proud of my Kayla. She bravely listened, asked a few questions, and seemed to understand far beyond what should be expected of a twelve year old. And she hugged me tightly, despite the tubes and wires.

I had been with Sarah Grace every single day of her young life until this awful time, and I missed her terribly. I worried that she would wonder why I hadn't come home to her, knowing she couldn't really understand that I was very sick. I wanted to hold her and to tell her that I loved her, even though I couldn't be at home with her.

The nurses agreed to let my mom "sneak" Sarah Grace into my room for a few minutes during visiting hours. It was such a relief to see her, comfortable in Grandma's arms. Of course, I knew in my head that she was ok, but my heart needed to see her with my eyes. She had obviously been taken care of very well, and was doing fine, even though I hadn't been singing her to sleep at night. It felt so good to see her gorgeous blue eyes.

I don't know if she didn't recognize me or if she was just afraid, but she didn't want to sit on the bed with me. I was lying down, totally flat, with wires and tubes in me, and no visible smile on my face. A big smile is what people my entire life had told me they most associated with me. Sarah Grace was probably worried when she saw me not smiling. I didn't have the strength to sit up or to hold her. I understood. It was ok. I was just so happy to see her. Greg's Caring Bridge entry that day said in part, *"Wenesday's mom and Kayla were able to get Sarah Grace into the ICU today for a short visit. I am certain that her heart has been warmed and her spirit strengthened with seeing Sarah Grace."*

The burning in my body had become unbearable. It felt like someone stabbed me in the back, right between my shoulder blades, with a knife, and then shot flames of hot fire from that hole in my back throughout every inch of my body, all the way to my toes and my fingers. I begged God to make the pain stop. I begged Him to let me sit, stand, walk, open and close my eyes normally, and to be able to hold my children and go home to them. I pleaded for the burning to stop, for mercy.

At that time, torture of prisoners of war was a big story in the news. I kept imagining that what I was feeling was probably very similar to what they were feeling. It was such awful pain. I thought though that it must be worse for them. What was happening to me was just a random thing. It just happened, and nobody knew why. What happened to people in war was inflicted upon them by other human beings. I imagined that would have to be much worse. I was thankful that I KNEW that everyone who knew me – and even many people who didn't know me – were wanting, hoping, and praying for the best for me. Nobody did this to me on purpose.

Still, I couldn't help but wonder why this was happening to me and to my family. One of my favorite nurses was a man named Tony. He was both knowledgeable and kind. Sarah Grace's name had sparked a conversation about southern double names, and he confided in me that his family called him Tony Bob, but everyone in the hospital simply knew him as Tony. Of course, I referred to him affectionately from that moment on as Tony Bob. His arms were covered in tattoos of crosses. He told me once that he had prayed for me. I asked him, "Tony Bob, why is this happening to me? Am I bad person?" He very seriously answered, "I don't know why this is happening to you. I don't think you're a bad person. Do you think you're a bad person?" I assured him that I did not think I was a bad person. When I discussed it with Greg, he said, "I don't know why this is happening to you either. It might be that one day, the purpose of this will be revealed. It might be that we will never know. Regardless, we can know that there is a reason."

I'm not a religious zealot. I wasn't raised going to church. My parents were hippies and told me that they wanted me to learn about all religions and make my own choice about what religion, if any, I wanted to belong to when I grew up. I was taught to love, to be kind and generous, and to treat others as I would like them to treat me.

I was exposed to many cultures and many religions as a child. Living in the Philippines, I saw Catholic families marching along the road on Easter Sunday. Men's heads were covered with pointy vines, and their hands were attached (some were tied and many were actually nailed) to huge, wooden crosses. The men would carry the heavy crosses on their backs and walk as their family members whipped them. I saw blood dripping down their backs.

We visited Japan and stayed in a Buddhist temple. We weren't allowed to wear shoes inside the temple, the interior walls were made of rice paper, and one of the monks gave me an umbrella to keep when it was raining. In Scotland, I took a religion class in school, which provided a basic overview of the main religions of the world, including Christianity. I noted that they all seemed to have a common theme – to leave the world a better place, to not kill other humans, to follow the rules that allow people to thrive. Those were the days before I knew anything about Islamic extremism, before 9/11/01.

My freshman year in college, a blonde haired, blue eyed, six year old boy named Henry died. I loved Henry – he had been so full of life and love. Henry was funny; he was mischievous, but not malicious. He wasn't a strict rule follower, but had not a mean bone in his tiny body. He always smiled, and truly cared about his friends. As a camp counselor for many summers, we weren't supposed to have teacher's pets, but Henry was my favorite kid each year. He was one of the regulars who returned each summer.

Henry had a heart condition that required him to have an internal pacemaker. I didn't know all of the details of what had gone on with him medically, but I had been told that he had a normal life expectancy. He simply had some minor needs for activity modifications. Sometimes, we'd go on long bear hunts during summer camp, hiking through the woods to see what animals we could spot. Henry would get winded, and I'd hoist him on my back. I didn't mind carrying him a bit, wanting him to enjoy the experience like all of our other campers.

Henry wasn't supposed to go under water while swimming. I don't know why, but it was a rule. His parents wanted him to enjoy the pool, so part of my job was to make sure he didn't push those limits. Surrounded by kids going under water, that was hard for him. More than once, he'd say, "Ms. Wenesday, remind me not to go underwater. I have wires in me." I'd smile and oblige.

I was sitting in my dorm room at LSU and Tara's quivering voice on the other end of the phone said, "Henry died. He was in a routine surgery and died on the operating table. Nobody had expected it." My eyes filled with tears. I ran across the hall and grabbed Betsy's Bible. She had grown up going to church and she knew the Bible from cover to cover. I threw it to her, crying hysterically, and said, "You show me where it says in here that a six year old should die!" That was the beginning of my real desire to learn about and become involved in Christianity, God, and

Jesus. After that, I began visiting different churches, trying to figure out where I belonged.

It was a long process. By the time I met Greg, I had been attending a Methodist church in Louisiana fairly regularly, thanks in large part to my good friend, Gina. Greg was a member of a nondenominational Christian church, but he agreed to go to the Methodist church with Kayla and me. I felt welcomed and comfortable there, and the sun shining in through the beautiful stained glass windows filled me with a good feeling of spirituality.

When Greg, Kayla, and I moved to the shiny brass buckle of America's Bible belt that is Jackson, TN, it was a change from anywhere I'd ever lived before. I have always been envious of all of the people for whom religion comes easily and naturally, for whom trying really wasn't necessary. When raised in a religious culture, born into a Christian heritage, it seems that there are easy and comforting answers to many of life's hard questions. When something horrible and unexpected happens, there is a reason. When something wonderful happens, there is a place to give praise and thanks. It seemed almost everyone in Jackson had that blessing.

People in Jackson, like all people, are human, capable of making good choices and susceptible to making mistakes. What sets this group of people apart in my view is that through it all, they maintain an unwavering faith. While many people put LSU or Yale signs in their yards to show their team affiliations, it's common in Jackson to see Jesus signs in people's yards.

What happened to me next was certainly a spiritual awakening, a hug from God. I had gone to our nondenominational Christian church the Sunday before being hospitalized, and the sermon was on Ezekiel 10. I had not read that part of the Bible before, but it now was clear that there had been a reason for me to hear that sermon that day. Part of the scripture reads, *"Then one of the cherubim reached out his hand to the fire that was among them. He took up some of it and put it into the hands of the man in linen, who took it and went out."*

The burning that was coursing through my veins that hurt a thousand times more than anything I'd ever experienced transformed. I saw a vision in my head of a winged creature of God who was on fire. That fire I saw in my mind became the fire burning through my body. The painful fire transformed into God's fire, and I found strength. I felt cleansed and revived. The burning became a good and tolerable burning. The pain did not stop; it was simply transformed into something good, worthy, and doable. God made it possible for me to endure.

I was overcome by an overwhelming feeling of peace. My life, which I had been reliving in memories, was amazing. I couldn't smile physically, but I was beaming internally. It was clear to me that I had smiled more in my thirty eight years than most people smile in their entire lifetimes. I had experienced so much good.

I had a loving family – parents who adored me and showered me with a life abundant in love, learning, and compassion. I had lived in three countries and visited many others. I had met and befriended an untold number of amazing people around the world, all from different cultures and backgrounds, and all good people.

9/11, a day and subsequent season of grief that had affected all Americans, had occurred in my lifetime. I was not in New York, but that day touched me. Kayla had been three years old, and I remembered explaining to her that bad guys had attacked our country, and that the good guys always win. I'd given her a twenty dollar bill to hand to a fireman collecting donations. She gave the hero the money and said with a smile, "this is for the good guys!"

I had lived through Hurricane Katrina. Kayla, Greg, my parents, Greg's mom, and I were evacuated from our Louisiana and Mississippi homes for well over a month. I had seen people suffer. I'd witnessed tears flow uncontrollably as people learned for the first time that their homes were under water, Greg's mom included. I had seen people help strangers, even at the risk of their own lives. I was privileged to have the honor of shaking the hands of some of the National Guardsmen who were working out of our Alexandria, LA hotel to fly missions, rescuing people from rooftops. I met an elderly man who worked in our hotel, who it appeared had very little himself, offering evacuees firm handshakes, hugs, smiles, clothes, food, and suggestions of free outings to allow kids to escape the depressing news suffocating the hotel lobby. We took Kayla to the Children's Museum in Alexandria on his advice.

The greater New Orleans area was a sad place, in mourning, for a long time. Many people lost loved ones, pets, homes, businesses, cars, and all possessions instantaneously. There were stories of ordinary people turned heroes swimming into windows to rescue elderly people trapped in their water-filled homes. A lot of the ER visits following the hurricane were actually from injuries people sustained with chainsaws while cutting tree limbs to help others access their homes.

When we returned home, it was like a scene from a movie. Our entire street, our entire neighborhood, was completely covered in tree branches and debris. Because of the chaos and the mayhem happening just across the bridge in New Orleans, there were signs written in permanent markers on large pieces of cardboard at the end of every street in our neighborhood that read, "You loot; we shoot."

Our yard stood out against the background of all of the rest. It was almost pristine. There was a levee (hill) of debris piled in front of it, making our grass lawn totally visible. Robin, my now sister-in-law, had cleaned up our yard (without telling us) so that Kayla wouldn't be afraid or sad when we got home. For that, I will be forever grateful. What a selfless act and an awesome gift!

I was thankful, humbled, and awed at the love I felt for my daughters. Kayla and Sarah Grace are the best things that have ever happened in my life. I was blessed with the most amazing daughters, beautiful inside and out. I had given birth to my girls, and I had gained my son, Ryan, through marriage vows to Greg. Ever since I could remember, I had always wanted three children. In adulthood, it seemed that wouldn't happen. Eventually, I was given three children who were absolutely perfect.

I have a master's degree in rehabilitation counseling and had worked full-time before and after becoming Kayla's mom. I liked my job, and loved its flexibility, but my child was always my priority, and it was often difficult to juggle everything. Greg had granted me the unbelievable gift of being a full-time mom to Kayla when we moved to Tennessee, and then to both Kayla and Sarah Grace after Sarah Grace was born.

I had experienced working outside of the home motherhood and full-time motherhood. I had seen my girls take their first steps. I had seen Kayla blossom into an incredible young lady – overflowing with love, kindness, intelligence, compassion, and humor. I had heard Sarah Grace giggle, had seen her readily share her toys at a very young age, felt her genuine hugs, and knew that even if I didn't live to see it, she was destined to spread happiness throughout the world with her kind and generous spirit.

My life was complete. While I wanted to live more of it and meet my future grandchildren, I felt at total peace. I knew that I had been blessed with an awesome life and that my family would be fine without me. I knew that Kayla would be alright. She was strong and would continue to bloom. I knew that she would always remember me with smiles and always know that I loved her. I knew that Kayla's father would allow her to continue her relationships with Greg and Sarah Grace and my parents, something that had consumed me with worry only hours earlier. I knew that Sarah Grace would grow and learn to understand that I didn't mean to leave her, and know that I loved her. I knew that together, Greg, Kayla, my mom, and my dad would instill in Sarah Grace some of my essence. I knew that Greg was an amazing father. I knew Sarah Grace would be ok.

I knew Greg would survive. He's internally the strongest man I've ever met. I knew he'd meet someone else one day who would help him raise our children, but I knew he would always remember and always love me, and he would always know I loved him. I knew we'd all one day be reunited in Heaven.

I knew with complete certainty that everything was going to be ok. It was all good. I had no loose ends in my life that needed to be tied. "Please, God, don't let me die" was replaced with, "Ok, God, my life is in your hands. If you want it to be time for me to leave this Earth, I'm ready. I'll embrace with open arms your plan for me and for my family, whatever it is. Thank you, God, for my awesome life. I couldn't have dreamed of a better one. I love you." I felt total peace.

Chapter 11

Hope, Hard Work, Pain, the Torture Chair

Almost immediately after I stopped fighting and put it all in God's hands, things started to take an unexpected turn for the better. Dr. Misulis wouldn't yet confirm for Greg that I had reached a plateau, but he did say that I hadn't deteriorated, and he actually sounded optimistic. Greg asked his familiar, "Has she reached the plateau yet?" Dr. Misulis' answer was out of the ordinary. This time, he responded, "I can't say with certainty she has reached the plateau, but I do see that for the first time since she's been in the hospital, her vital signs did not worsen overnight. She seems to be a little bit stronger. We are not out of the woods yet, but I am encouraged by what I'm seeing." God wanted me to live. I was back in the fight for my life. It wasn't going to be easy, but it was so worth it.

Dr. Misulis' newest concern though was that all of the horizontal living I was doing was causing problems for my lungs. He wanted me to get vertical, even though it would be passively, since I still couldn't move on my own volition. Having the bed raised even thirty degrees caused excruciating nerve pain.

Dr. Misulis got creative. He thought that perhaps if he moved me out of the hospital bed and into a "stroke chair" – a cushioned, reclining chair – it would make getting somewhat vertical easier on me. I readily agreed. I was eager to try anything that would get me out of the bed and that would hasten my recovery. It was decided on a

Friday that the new exercise would take place the next day. I was actually pretty excited.

On Saturday morning, the lift team arrived in my room. A nurse told my dad, who had been visiting me, "I'm going to have to ask you to leave now so we can get Wenesday sitting up in this chair." We were a little surprised that he'd have to leave, but didn't question it. My dad kissed my forehead and told me he would return the next day. I was disconnected from the tubes and wires and beeping machines.

The lift team consisted of four strong men whose goal was to move me by holding the sheet I was lying on and carrying the sheet taut with me in it across my room from the bed to the chair. As soon as they lifted me, my body was no longer still and flat, but moving in the sheet wherever gravity took it. With that movement came indescribable pain. I knew instantly this was a bad idea. "Never mind! I don't want to do this anymore! This hurts! I don't want to do this! Put me back in my bed! PLEASE!" The lift team looked toward the nurse, who instructed them to continue on the journey.

I was laid down in the chair. Ouch! Oh, my God! Fire shot from the knife that felt lodged between my shoulder blades, down to my toes, and out to my fingertips. It was unbearable. I cried loudly. I pleaded with the nurse to return me to the flat bed. He told me that he was sorry, but that it was for my own good.

St. Thomas – our wedding – I tried to visualize it – I tried to escape – but it didn't work. I pulled out the big guns. I pictured the birth of Kayla and the birth of Sarah Grace – the two happiest days of my life. I clenched my eyes as tightly as I could and tried to focus on my girls' faces, their eyes. Oh, the pain! The fire! My visualization escape wasn't working. I focused on breathing. I focused on God's fire. Nothing was helping. It hurt so badly.

All I could think about was when I had my babies, I had epidurals. I called for the nurse and pleaded with him to give me an epidural. I knew that would work at least somewhat. I knew there was such medicine in that hospital, because I had one when Sarah Grace was born in that very building. The nurse explained that I already had pain medicine in my body, and then said words that I will never in my life forget, "Darlin', we don't have any medicine in this hospital strong enough to take away the kind of pain you have. You have nerve pain."

I was assured again that the torture was for my own good and would last only fifteen minutes. The nurse had instructed the lift team to return after fifteen minutes. Those were definitely the longest and hardest minutes of my life. There was no escape; this was torture I was going to have to endure. Through blurry, tear-filled eyes, I watched the second hand on the wall clock slowly tick away.

The nurse and the lift team were true to their word. After exactly fifteen minutes, they were all back in my room and looking at me compassionately. They returned me to my flat bed using the previous transport method and reattached the tubes and wires. I had endured. I had survived.

It took some time for the pain to subside and for me to return to my new normal level of "comfort." I was given more pain medicine. I was told we would do it again the next day. I asked to speak to Dr. Misulis or Liz, knowing neither of them would want me to suffer the level of pain that this procedure had caused. It was the weekend though, and neither would return until Monday.

My mom, my best friend, is a very strong, resilient woman who regularly makes lemonade out of lemons. She does tend to get emotional though, especially regarding me, her only child. I instinctively knew that I had to protect my mom, not share with her the depths of my pain or my fears. I told her some things and sugar coated other things to the best of my ability. She was my mom, and I was, even as an adult, her baby. I put on a strong show for her, knowing that as a mom myself, I would not be able to handle watching my child suffer. When she visited and asked me about the chair, I simply said, "It wasn't fun."

My dad was tough though. He had been a marine in Viet Nam. He had been injured and received a Purple Heart, and he never discussed it. He was almost never emotional. He had been my rock of strength my whole life, able to handle anything that came our way. When we lived in the Philippines, we had to have typhoid and cholera shots. One of those shots had to be injected into the arm muscle, not just the skin surface, and hurt quite a bit. My dad got his first. He had an allergic reaction, which caused nurses and doctors to move hurriedly and draw circles on his arm to monitor the swelling. He stood there with a brave smile plastered on his face, telling me it was no big deal, being a tough role model, knowing my mom's and my arms would be the next to receive the shots.

We were at the beach one day, in the ocean, and some girls alerted my friend and me that there were jellyfish in the area. Brandi and I took off running toward the sandy beach. Before we reached it, Brandi was stung, fell down, and started crying. My dad ran into the beautiful Subic Bay saltwater and scooped my friend up into his arms. As he stood holding her on the sandy beach, the lifeguards tended to the tiny sting on her leg. Suddenly, my mom let out a shriek, noticing that my dad had a huge jellyfish tentacle wrapped all the way around his leg. Only then did the lifeguards pull off the tentacle and treat his skin, where there would later be a scar that looked like barbed wire had wrapped around his leg. That had to sting, but he hadn't said a word, making sure the crying little girl was cared for first.

When my dad visited me the following day, I told him I was going to be placed in the torture chair again. He asked, "I wonder why they made me leave yesterday?" I detailed for him what it had been like. As I described the pain, my voice cracked and tears flowed. "It hurt, Dad; it hurt like I've never felt anything hurt before. It felt like someone put a knife between my shoulder blades and shot flames out from the knife. I felt the burning first in my back, then down into my legs and toes, then through my arms and into my hands. I felt like I was being set on fire from the inside out. I don't think I can do it again. I know I need to sit, but I can't. Please don't let them do that to me again."

I had never before in my life seen my dad's face contort the way it did then. He was holding back tears. My 6'4" tall, muscular, tough guy of a dad with a bulldog tattoo on his bicep and a very deep voice, afraid of nothing, was suddenly reduced to simply being a vulnerable dad whose daughter was suffering, knowing that nothing he could do could take away her pain. He quietly nodded his head in understanding and said, "That's why they made me leave. I couldn't have handled that." I think my dad aged twenty years before my eyes in that one moment. Even his hair genuinely looked grayer.

I knew then that my dad had to be protected too. Greg would be my rock. He could carry the reality of the pain I would have to endure on his shoulders. He had to.

Greg was not only my rock, but my advocate too – my liaison to the medical staff, and he would fight for my best interests. Every time he walked into my room, I felt better. This time, I KNEW he would understand that the suffering was too much, that I could not be moved to that chair again. I knew he would put a stop to it.

Our yin and yang resurfaced. Greg's response was true to his type A "when the going gets tough, the tough get going" personality. He is the most compassionate person I know, but also believes in hard work and suffering for the greater good. He didn't support the chair to be mean; he did it because he truly believed it was the best thing for me at that moment. "Dr. Misulis said it's vital for you to sit up in the chair. I know you don't want to do it. I understand it hurts. You want to get better and get home to Kayla and Sarah Grace, don't you? Wenesday, you have to sit in the chair. You can do this. I know you can. You will get through it. You are strong." Greg, with empathy and love, had told me I needed to endure the torture chair again on Sunday, and I did.

I knew that if Greg thought it was good for me, it most likely was, but that was bitter medicine to swallow. If I had been able to write, my Caring Bridge post would have said something to the effect of, *"This is awful. No human should have to endure the pain I am suffering. I wouldn't wish this on my worst enemies. I want to go home. I want to walk. I want to hold my one year old baby in my arms. I want to hug my twelve year old girl. I want to be a wife to my husband. Does anyone know how to stop this pain, both physically and emotionally? Someone, please help me!"*

I couldn't write though, and fortunately, never did send such a pitiful note. Greg's Caring Bridge post on Monday morning said, in part, *"Wenesday had another good night on Saturday and Sunday as the Lord continues to show His greatness. We are confident that she has hit the plateau of GBS even though the doctor hasn't used those words yet. He again stated that he 'sees some improvement' and he is 'encouraged' by her progress thus far. The pulmonologist has stated that her lungs are improving and her lung capacity has been relatively good. The cardiologist will discontinue his rounds because her heart is strong. She does still continue to experience significant pain when they require her to sit in a chair, and as much as I hate to say it, the pain is good for her (sorry, Wenesday)...her spirits are good...."*

Chapter 12

Messages of Hope (Positive Energy)

Throughout my hospital stay, every time Greg visited, the first thing he did was read Caring Bridge posts to me. I looked forward to hearing them. They kept me connected to people outside of the hospital walls, encouraged me, and often made me laugh.

People always said I had a unique sense of humor, and I had always been known for and prided myself on being an optimist. Julie wrote, *"I really miss your smiling face, unstoppable attitude and quirky yet charming and joyful outlook on life...."*

Jennifer had always seemed to share my quirky sense of humor. She wrote, *"I know your crazy, fiery spirit and positive attitude will see you through this so we can get back to planning Sarah Grace and Garrett's wedding."* Garrett was Jennifer's one year old son and Sarah Grace's first boyfriend.

While I also missed my smiling face, I focused on what Julie and Jennifer – who didn't even know each other, and lived in different states – had both said about my attitude. I quickly realized that it was a good thing this was happening to me and not to a negative person. If it got me down, I could only imagine what it would do to someone who wasn't generally happy. It was a good thing it was me. I could handle it. With my optimism, I could handle anything that came my way! I truly appreciated that reminder from my friends. It became a common theme in people's posts.

Doc, our friend who was going through serious medical issues himself, selflessly posted at 2:17 in the morning, *"As you can see, it's another sleepless night for me, so I'll put it to good use by praying for a speedy recovery for you...."* Even people fighting their own health battles were taking the time to pray and care for me. That was humbling.

Hunter, my old college buddy who exemplifies fun and has not a serious bone in his body, wrote, *"I am so sad to hear about your illness. I am not a very religious man, but this situation calls for a special prayer to the Big Guy upstairs. I wish you a speedy recovery and strength for your family! Know that everyone is pulling for your recovery! If only you would have eaten meat all those years! Just kidding, but seriously – get better! The world needs more people like you with your great smile and good heart!"* I used to call my friend Gatherer, not acknowledging that he was named after one who killed animals. Hunter was a good guy. If my sickness prompted him to talk to God for the first time in a long time, that had to be a good thing. His post made me smile internally.

I have an addiction to taking – and sharing – photographs. People tend to complain as I photograph them, but later appreciate having the mementos. My friend, Sandra, nicknamed me years ago a documatrix. I even made that my Halloween costume one year. I had a film whip. She wrote, *"Glad to hear you are having a better day today. I miss your documatrix updates! Praying for your full and speedy recovery!"* I had been off of social media since entering the hospital. I hadn't even taken any pictures – unheard of for me.

Gina posted, *"Think of this verse daily: Philippians 4:13 – 'I can do all things through Christ who strengthens me.' God will carry you through this and with your motivation and perseverance I know He will have an easier job!"* All of my doctors and therapists had commented on how hard I worked and fought. It was rewarding hearing Gina's words.

I have always loved Julie's cooking. She wrote, *"Thinking of you today as I cook for a girls' bunko night. You'd be proud of me; I have lots of vegetarian options! Roasted tomato soup with focaccia, goat cheese rolled in pistachios and dried cranberries, Greek salad, pecan pie tarts...and a little grilled meat for those who partake in animal flesh. Your smiling face would be a wonderful addition around the table! Hang in there, darling, and I'm praying for you daily."* Julie's cooking sounded better than the liquid that was being pumped into me through a tube. The weird thing though was that I didn't have any appetite. I really wasn't hungry.

Aubrey's description made me proud, and her meat comments brought me to laughter, *"You're such a strong, happy, vivacious woman who's always up for everything and so full of life. You leave such a positive and heart-warming effect on everyone who has the privilege to meet you. Praying for a speedy recovery so you can get back to cooking some vegetarian meals for that family of yours! I'm sure they're miserable having to eat meat three meals a day. I miss you!"* It was true that my family was eating better with me in the hospital than they ever had, thanks to our army of friends.

Tara wrote, *"I think about you nearly every minute and am sending all the good energy, positive vibes, love and prayers out to you. With your positive attitude, your body has no choice but to follow the example you've set and get on with the business of healing! I can't wait to see your smiling face again! We ALL love you so very much! We are with you every minute, even if not in person. Your courage and strength inspires me. Keep up the fight because you're winning! Take one day at a time. Right now you just have to get through today; when that seems impossible, know that I'm just a phone call away."* Tara's words brought warmth to my heart. The nurses said we could bend the rules and keep my phone in my room. The problem was that my vision was too blurry for me to text or dial, and my voice was too weak to talk.

I was in a service organization, Jackson Service League, and enjoyed participating in Children's Theater, which allowed us to put on plays for children who might not otherwise ever see live theater. It took a lot of time. Taylor made me smile with, *"Ashley told me about the great lengths you are taking to get out of Children's Theater. I do think this is a bit extreme. I would have helped...."* She also offered that her husband, a physician who worked in the hospital, could translate medical jargon and visit outside of visiting hours. I appreciated that. I had never realized before just how many friends I had who worked in the hospital.

My dear friend, Karen, who is Scottish and lives in England, wrote, *"What are you up to scaring us all? I so wish I could be there for you, but the Atlantic is unfortunately in our way. You need to start getting better so you can start planning the St. Thomas reunion next year...."* Karen was one of my best friends when I lived in Scotland. She had come to St. Thomas for Greg's and my wedding. We had planned on a five year anniversary trip. The prospect of that anniversary trip was exciting; the reality that it now may not happen was disheartening. The fact that Karen was thinking of me from the other side of the ocean was heartwarming, and brought to life for me the fact that I truly did have people pulling for me all over the world.

I missed the school musical Kayla was in for the first time ever. Carol wrote, *"Just wanted to report that Kayla and company did great in Aladdin last night. Super fantastic show! I snapped a few pics that I will tag on your Facebook page. I want you to feel a part of it...."* I had shed many a tear missing that play, and wondering what else I would miss. It felt good to know that once again, my army of friends was stepping in to help make things better.

Jennifer could always make me laugh, *"I had a surprise last night. When I was checking a voice mail, a message you had left before getting sick popped up instead. It was one of your super long, marathon messages that I can wash a whole sink full of dishes to. It was wonderful to hear your voice. I know how much you miss leaving those messages and I miss hearing them terribly. I hope tonight is another small step and your toughness holds. I have decided not to do any more dishes until you are out! Love you all!"* I had to hurry and get better. Jennifer's family couldn't eat on dirty dishes because of me!

Eventually, after I returned home, I printed and bound the Caring Bridge pages. There are one hundred nineteen of them. Every word brought me internal smiles, reminded me how many people were in my corner, and added immensely to my strength. I am thankful from the bottom of my heart to all who added to this treasure that I will keep forever.

Chapter 13

Dreams and Progress

I had the most wonderful, glorious, vivid dream of my life while in the NICU. It felt so real, yet in reality, seemed so far out of reach. It was so simple, yet so amazing. In my dream, I was RUNNING through the hospital hallways, leaping like a gazelle. I was squealing in delight and smiling so big that none of the doctors or nurses who'd only known my paralyzed face recognized me. It was pure joy. Then, I awoke…and told everyone I could about it.

I had planned to tell Dr. Misulis and Liz Monday morning about how the torture chair had affected my body and to plead my case to not have to endure it again. I understood the no pain, no gain mantra, but I also knew the difference between good pain and bad pain. The chair caused bad pain. I knew it was more harmful to me than good, and I knew I could convince them.

My neurologist and physical therapist entered my room together. Before I could utter a word, they related to me that the nurses had told them about my experiences in the chair and they had agreed that I would not be subjected to that again. I let out a huge sigh of relief! They had a new plan. Liz would bring her strongest helper and she and he would work with me, at a pace I could tolerate, slowly and gently, to sit on the side of the bed with support. I was skeptical, but hopeful, and quickly agreed. Anything would be better than the torture chair.

Early on, when Liz had first started working with me, she had taped a piece of paper behind my bed so that caregivers and visitors could see the exercises that I was supposed to do and help me do them as often as possible. They included such things as someone moving my legs up and down and out to the sides and rotating my ankles for me. Liz had tied yellow stretchy bands to my bed rails and instructed me to do bicep curls with them to help prevent any further decline in my upper body strength. I had asked her if she could tape the instructions to the TV in front of me, so that I could see them and do what I could. She said I was the first person to ever show her such initiative from the NICU bed. I worked tirelessly on those bicep curls. Liz knew I was trying to get better, and I loved that she seemed to go above and beyond to help me.

Prior to becoming a full-time mom, I had spent about eleven years working as a vocational rehabilitation case manager. Most of my clients were in the workers' compensation system. Many of them clearly genuinely wanted to get better. I enjoyed working with those people. Unfortunately, some of my clients seemed to have gotten comfortable being paid to not work, and didn't appear to put much effort into their rehabilitation. Those clients caused me some frustration. I understood better than most people that a positive attitude and hard work would lead to a stronger outcome and faster finish. I wanted to be the star patient, working as hard as I could, getting to return home strong with minimal limitations.

Liz appeared in my room with a large, muscular man. He was over six feet tall and solid. He gave me a huge bear hug and answered my fearful tears with confidence. He looked straight into my eyes and said, "God bless you! I promise you I will not drop you! I won't let you fall!" I let the two of them pull my torso upright and move me to the edge of the bed. I had no trunk control at all – I was totally in their hands. While I trusted them, the idea of falling onto the floor and breaking bones could not be shaken.

The act of being put into a seated position caused the expected pain, but I was determined. This was a gentler and safer way of doing what was necessary to bring me one step closer to going home to my family. We watched the clock with the goal of me sitting, fully supported of course, for one minute. I talked to Liz through the pain and far surpassed our original goal. I was proud!

Greg's Caring Bridge entry from that day said in part, *"In lieu of the 'pain chair,' they are allowing her to gradually sit up on the side of the bed. Today, she sat up for four minutes, which is excellent. Her PT is going well, and her arms and hands feel stronger. She was even able to send handwritten notes home to Kayla and Sarah Grace. She is working hard now to help reduce the amount of PT required later and aid in a rapid recovery. In general, she has more energy, strength, facial expression, eye contact and movement. Her recovery thus far is miraculous and we are thankful to our Father in Heaven for His mercy and faithfulness. Please continue to pray for her full and speedy recovery. In addition, please pray for her emotional strength as I know it is very difficult for her to be without her little Kayla and her little Sarah Grace and her doggies. Please pray for Kayla and Sarah Grace as well; they miss their mommy. Keep the Caring Bridge guestbook entries coming and keep visiting, these are the highlights of her days. We love you, Wenesday!"*

Chapter 14

Transitions

On my eleventh day in the hospital, Dr. Misulis walked into my NICU room and said two sentences that will forever be etched in my memory, "This room is reserved for really sick patients only. We are going to have to kick you out." I was being sprung from the NICU with promises of my family and friends and even youngest daughter being able to visit my next room with no regard for the clock. YES! I was overjoyed! I was on the road to recovery and normalcy. I had worked hard, and was proud of myself. I had prayed hard, and was thankful to God. I was elated that visible progress was finally being made.

Many of my doctors and nurses came to tell me good bye before I left my NICU room. I loved them all for caring enough to take time out of their busy schedules to visit me and wish me well. I felt like we had become close during my stay. There is a psychological term for feeling an emotional bond with care takers, but this was real. We had laughed, cried, made small talk, and they had kept me alive. I would be forever grateful for their part in my recovery, for all they had done for me.

Some of them warned me that while the transfer was good news, what was to come would not be a cakewalk. I was warned that the around the clock care I had been accustomed to would be less frequent, but the good news was that it would be that way because I was strong enough to no longer need medical staff at my side every second of the day. They all encouraged me; wished me strength during the next phase of my hospital stay; and cheered me on, saying they had faith that I would thrive. They also reminded me that while help wouldn't be visible through a window in my room, as it had been, it still wasn't far away. I was told to always ask for help when I needed it.

A friendly transport worker pushed me, still horizontal in my bed, to my new room on the regular floor. My stuff – cards, cell phone, disposable toothbrushes, notebook, etc. – was placed into a bag and onto my bed to make the short and happy journey with me.

My new "regular" room was smaller, but it didn't really matter because I couldn't get out of bed. My room was next to the nurse's station. I couldn't see the nurses, but I could sometimes hear them, and I knew they were there. My new nurses greeted me with smiles. I was even treated to a familiar face – one of the NICU nurses was filling in on my new floor. I still had a feeding tube, I still couldn't sit on my own, and I still couldn't stand at all.

The biggest change with the new room was that it came without visiting hours. My family and friends were able to come with no regard to the slowly ticking second hand on the wall clock. That was wonderful. Greg instructed Stephanie that her most important nanny duty was to take Sarah Grace to the hospital to visit me daily while he was at work and Kayla was in school. He also asked Stephanie to be sure Sarah Grace had a pretty bow in her hair daily, something that made me happy. Liz and some of the nurses who hadn't been on duty when I was transferred out of the NICU came to visit me throughout the day in my new room. I truly felt cared about, and not just like a generic hospital patient. My speech was beginning to gradually improve, so even though I couldn't smile at all, people were starting to understand me more easily.

The next day, Liz appeared at my door with a wheelchair. It was time for me to sit up and work on regaining some independence. While I was fully aware that it would hurt, I was very eager and excited to try. Liz and a helper picked me up and placed me in the wheelchair. It hurt a lot. She exchanged the chair for one with a taller back and propped a pillow behind me for added support and comfort, which helped a little. I pushed myself! It was funny because while both of my arms were weak, one was stronger than the other, and I did not move in a straight line. I ran my wheelchair crooked, right into the wall. One might think that would be disheartening; however, it jived well with my goofy sense of humor. I thought it was hilarious and laughed.

It felt good to be able to propel myself in a wheelchair – good enough to be able to deal with the pain in my back caused by being in a sitting position. I knew this was a huge accomplishment, and I was beaming internally. I had a group of cheerleaders – people who'd helped me in the hospital and were genuinely happy to see this progress – and my hubby, of course - clapping loudly for me! Greg's Caring Bridge entry that day said, *"Today, Wenesday made it into a wheelchair and was able to move herself about 35 feet! Amazing!"*

Later that day – it was a big day – I was taken downstairs for a swallowing test in order to ascertain whether or not it was safe for the feeding tube to be removed and for me to be given food orally. I was nervous about the test and about the fact that I would have to remain in a seated position throughout it with people who were not physical therapists and might not understand my difficulty with being upright. Liz offered to accompany me. It wasn't part of her normal scope of duties – it was yet another above and beyond moment that she gave me. I was thankful.

She waited with me until it was my turn, and then talked to the professionals who were giving me the swallowing test on my behalf. I was strapped into a chair so I wouldn't fall over, and I had to sit completely vertical. I had to swallow tiny bits of liquids and foods while people watched it go through my system on an X-ray in order to be sure it wasn't entering the wrong pipe and going into my lungs. I was told I did well and could be free of the feeding tube possibly in just a few days.

A new care taker introduced herself to me – a rehabilitation specialist named Dr. Payne. The irony of her name was not lost when she talked about transferring me to the rehabilitation unit. She began, "I love your name. Wenesday is such a beautiful and unique name." I answered, "I hope your name isn't foreboding of what you're going to do to me. I guess with your last name, you were destined to be a physical medicine doctor." We both laughed.

Dr. Payne was honest. She said, "Rehabilitation is a big step forward, but I will warn you that it will probably be difficult and even painful. Most people choose to spend at least a few days in the regular room resting, after being released from the NICU, before moving to the rehabilitation floor. You are young. I have been told that you are strong and extremely motivated. The best results are obtained when people begin rehabilitation sooner rather than later. It is up to you if you want to move to the rehabilitation floor today or wait a few days."

I knew my recovery was going to be an uphill battle. I still had no movement in my legs. I knew I wanted to do everything in my power to get home to my family. I remembered from my days working as a rehabilitation counselor that there was truth in what she said about sooner rehabilitation leading to better outcomes. Of course, I opted to move that day.

When the transport team arrived, I had two visitors in my room. Christy gave me a hug, and Holly agreed to accompany me on my journey. The transport team insisted they had to take two oxygen canisters with me, as they had when I moved from the NICU to the regular room, even though I said I didn't need them. I was improving, not regressing. I was determined. They had to follow rules though, and the oxygen canisters made the journey with me in my bed while Holly walked next to us. Since my view was of the ceiling, I had no sense of direction, but after an elevator ride and many turns down different hallways, we arrived in my new room on the rehabilitation unit. Since I still had a feeding tube and a catheter and was still paralyzed and completely dependent on others, I was given the room directly across from the nurse's station.

My room had a fairly large window and I was grateful. It turned out that from my bed, when I looked to the left out the window, I was able to see the emergency helicopter land and take off in the distance. I couldn't see the entire view, but I was able to watch the tops of people's helmets running to and from the helicopter at all times of the day and night. It gave me something interesting to look at and it made me keenly aware that there were other people in the hospital in worse positions than me. I said a lot of prayers for those people, whoever they were.

We had been told that on the rehabilitation floor, I would be able to ditch the hospital gowns and wear my own clothes; specifically, comfortable exercise clothes. Greg had brought a bag of my clothes to the regular room. Holly unpacked them for me in my new rehabilitation room where I actually had a closet and small chest of drawers. I couldn't access them myself, but it felt good to have them in my room. It also felt good having a friend there helping me. Greg arrived as soon as he could and admired my new space.

A physical therapist named Mark entered my room. Mark was friendly and knowledgeable. He explained that he wouldn't be my regular PT, but that he was going to do my introduction and evaluation. My regular PT would be back at work Monday morning. Mark was Filipino American, and I told him I had lived in the Philippines for four years as a child. Our rapport came easily and he seemed very caring. He even told me that he was a pastor in his church, and that he would pray for me.

Mark had to review the rules of the rehabilitation floor with me. "In order to benefit from being allowed to participate in this intense program that you need, and not get kicked out early by your insurance company, you must strictly adhere to the rules. You are required to attend all of your sessions. Guess why most people who miss their sessions miss them? It's because they're in the bathroom. Plan ahead. Going to the bathroom is not considered a valid excuse for missing therapy."

Mark said that PT would be hard and that I might even cry, but that it would be well worth it. They would work my body in order to help it regain its strength. I was not to take pictures in the therapy room due to privacy concerns of other patients. I was not to accept phone calls or visitors during therapy. I had to show continued progress, even if in very small increments. If I plateaued and stopped improving at all, or when I improved to a point of being able to go home and benefit from less intense outpatient therapy, my insurance would stop paying and I would be discharged. He didn't know for sure, but speculated when I pressed him that I might stay on the rehabilitation floor for six weeks.

Mark did a physical evaluation. I closed my eyes while he poked various spots on my feet, legs, and ankles. I was supposed to tell him if he was pricking me with a sharp point or with something dull. Most of the time, it was hard for me to tell. It all felt the same. My feet were tingling, like they were defrosting from having been in the snow. I didn't know if the instrument was pointy or dull. He instructed me to guess. A couple times the touch hurt, and I reacted with a loud, "ouch." Sometimes, I couldn't feel his touch at all – I only knew he was touching me because he told me.

After the evaluation, he noted that my sensations were odd and confused, as is a hallmark of Guillain-Barre' syndrome. At one point, he barely touched me, and I cried out in pain. At another point, he was squeezing my ankle as hard as he could – said it would have made a grown man scream – and I wasn't even aware that he was touching me.

Mark asked if my house was wheelchair accessible. My house has one step outside leading to the front door. He asked if my husband would be able to build a ramp. Greg can build anything, I told him, but I wanted to go home walking. He said that he was hopeful I would return home ambulatory, but that we needed to be prepared for the possibility of going home in a wheelchair. While most do, not everyone with Guillain-Barre' can walk again.

That was a sobering pill to swallow, but I felt optimistic. I would beat the odds. I would beat this horrible thing called Guillain-Barre' Syndrome. I was tough, strong, determined, and had my family to fight for.

Flowers started arriving again and filled the shelves of my rehabilitation room from my first day there. They were beautiful, and the fact that so many people cared enough to send them so quickly made me feel good. I kept looking at them happily. Greg brought more pictures and my electric toothbrush for the counter. Kayla, Sarah Grace, and my parents visited. Everyone was excited for me. I was feeling good. I was feeling optimistic. Then, night fell on my first day in the rehabilitation unit.

Chapter 15

The Night Shift

In the "regular" room and in the rehabilitation room, the nurses and assistants would write their names on a dry erase board on my wall at the beginning of their shifts. I noticed that in previous rooms, there were nurses and aides. On the rehab floor, there were nurses and techs. I hadn't been in the rehab room a full day, but it appeared that the aides and techs basically did the same things. Being the grammar nerd I am, I was curious about the different titles.

When my Friday night shift tech entered my room for the first time, I very politely and with a friendly tone introduced myself. She barely looked my way. I asked her to pull up my covers (I physically could not do so myself). Until that moment, every person I'd encountered in the hospital happily helped me. She seemed irritated. I got the impression she wished I was asleep so she wouldn't have to deal with me.

I tried to make small talk. I asked her what the difference was between the titles. Her answer was anything but what I had expected to hear.

She said, "In the other units, the aides go to school and earn that title. In rehab, any person can walk in off the street and apply for a job with no training and be hired to be a tech. I am the only tech on this floor that went to school to become a tech. Everyone else here just walked in off the street without any training at all." With that, she pulled up my covers and left my room. I was taken aback.

My Friday night nurse introduced herself. She was pretty with blonde hair down her back and make up perfectly applied, she was happy and bubbly, she was young…very young. I asked and she told me she was twenty-one.

I was suddenly keenly aware that I had entered a different world. The people helping me in this new environment were young, inexperienced, much less friendly, and hurried, having to attend to a lot of other patients as well as me. I still couldn't sit or move my legs on my own. I still had to be turned regularly so I wouldn't get bed sores. I was anything but self-sufficient. It was dark, my family and friends were all at home tucked snugly in their beds, and I was all alone and suddenly very scared again.

At 3 AM, I awoke in pain and filled with anxiety. I called my young nurse. It took her longer to get to me than it had taken the nurses in the NICU or on the general floor, and when she arrived, I told her about my anxiety and pain. She looked at my chart and told me I had been asleep when it was time for my medications and nobody had awakened me. I asked to take them then. She said that my pain medicine and anxiety medicine were scheduled drugs and that if I missed a time, I would have to wait for the next scheduled time to get the medicine.

I politely argued that didn't make sense. I didn't want to take an extra dose; I simply wanted the medication prescribed by my physician a couple hours late because I had apparently slept through the scheduled time. She wouldn't budge. I was not given my medicine.

My excitement and enthusiasm for transferring to the rehab floor was being replaced with terror. Maybe I'd been overzealous. Maybe I wasn't ready yet. Maybe I should've stayed on the regular floor longer. What if I couldn't perform and was kicked out of the program before I'd received the full benefit from it?

I was having a panic attack. For the first time during my entire hospital stay, I didn't wait for the clock to tell me that the rest of the world was awake, but I called Greg at 3:00 or 4:00 in the morning. Fortunately, I had gained the finger dexterity and vision clarity to carefully and slowly push the necessary phone buttons to make a call to someone in my contact list. Greg listened compassionately, sounded appropriately worried, reassured me, and told me he would visit first thing in the morning. I reminded him that the dry erase board in my room showed that my schedule Saturday morning would be as follows:

7:00 – 8:30 AM Occupational Therapy (OT)

9:30 – 10:30 AM Physical Therapy (PT)

3:30 – 4:00 PM Physical Therapy (PT)

Saturday morning, my occupational therapist (OT) greeted me at the door with a friendly smile promptly at 7:00. Her name was Amy, and she exuded confidence and enthusiasm. I felt safe with her. She told me that our main order of business would be to get me bathed and dressed and my teeth brushed.

Before then, I had been given periodic sponge baths while lying in bed. This time, she sat me on the side of the bed with my feet dangling off the edge, and I was able to balance somewhat while holding on to the bed. She gave me the wet, soapy washcloth to bathe myself while she helped support me upright. I washed my face and the parts of me I could reach, and she got the rest. Then, she handed me my toothbrush and brought me a basin to spit into. I brushed my teeth by myself. She got me dressed for the most part, but I put my shirt over my head myself. This was the most I'd taken care of myself in almost two weeks, and it felt empowering! I was really happy with the progress.

As happy as I was, I was also exhausted and hurting. It had been a long night and a physically active (relative to what I'd become used to) morning. The same nurse who had skipped my overnight medicine visited after my OT session. I asked her if it was time for my medication, and she told me that the time had come and gone while the OT was working with me. She hadn't wanted to interrupt the session, and I had again missed the medicine schedule. I could not believe it.

Greg arrived at the hospital bright and early to give me a much needed tight hug. He was disturbed to hear the details about my medication, or lack thereof. His facial expression was very serious as he listened patiently. At that point, I had missed two doses of pain and anxiety medicine. I was crying uncontrollably. Greg said, "That is not acceptable. I am going to talk to Dr. Payne," and he left my room. Greg returned, followed by Dr. Payne.

I told her all about what had happened with the nurse and what the tech had said about them not being trained. Dr. Payne said sympathetically, "I am sorry that happened to you. That nurse is good, but new and inexperienced. She should have given you your medicine. She will receive additional training during her next shift. I will ask your current nurse to get your medicine right away." Dr. Payne also said that particular tech had been reprimanded for other things and had already been on thin ice. Dr. Payne assured me, "All of the techs on the rehabilitation floor have been thoroughly trained. I would trust them to take care of me and of my relatives. You are in good hands."

Although the move to the rehab floor represented progress, it marked a transition in the level of care I would receive. I only saw that initial tech one more time, and then never again. It was a week or so before I saw the young blonde nurse again, and when I did, she apologized for what had happened, and said that she now understood that I could get medicine that I had missed. The other nurses and techs on the rehab floor did turn out to be amazingly good, knowledgeable, and compassionate. I got to know them all. Before too long, I was able to trust them all completely.

Gerardo, my physical therapist (PT), was tall and originally from South America. He came to my room at 9:30 in the morning. I was initially eager and excited to get to work. "Are you ready to get started?" I answered enthusiastically, "I sure am! I want you to know that I am happy to do this, and I am smiling, even though my face isn't cooperating." Gerardo wheeled me to the gym to orient me to the room where I would receive physical therapy. When he showed me the parallel bars though and said, "You will walk with these bars soon," my mood began to shift from excitement to fear. "How will I do that? I can't move my legs at all." He said, "You will learn to support yourself with your arms, and your legs will eventually follow. I will be right behind you the whole time, keeping you steady."

Didn't he know my arms were weak? I couldn't lift myself with my arms alone. Surely, I would fall. I looked at my legs, trying to get them to move, but they wouldn't. They didn't even budge an inch. While looking down at my paralyzed legs, instead of movement, I saw a huge drop of water on my leg, followed by another one, and another one. One of the big drops rolled down my leg and hit the floor. It took me a minute to realize that what I was seeing was my tears. I was crying again. I am not usually a crier.

It had been a big day. Gerardo asked, "Why are you crying?" I wasn't really sure myself. "I think I'm scared. I'm not usually a baby like this. I'm tough. I can't walk on those bars though. I will fall and injure myself even worse if I try. My legs won't move at all. I know they won't support my weight. I really don't think I can do this. I'm afraid it's too soon."

Gerardo tried to reassure me. He told me, "We're not going to start with the bars. You will work your way up to using them. I was just showing them to you so you can look forward to it. You will be surprised at what you will accomplish in therapy. We will work together and you will get stronger. I will keep you safe, and I promise you I will not let you get hurt. We'll just call today an orientation day though, and wait to begin the work tomorrow."

Gerardo wheeled me back to my room and lifted me back into bed. I was physically and emotionally exhausted. Greg was waiting for me in my room with a listening ear, hugs, and love – the medicine I desperately needed at that moment. I felt like I had let the world down, being such a wimp. I had wanted to begin therapy; I hadn't anticipated the fear and anxiety I would experience. Greg quietly reassured me, "It is ok. You've had a long night and a big day. Today was your first day. You're doing great. I am proud of you."

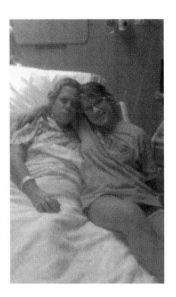

Here, I was snuggling with Kayla, so of course, I was smiling big on the inside. I'd hoped a closed mouth smile might show a little better, but it didn't. It looked like a frown on the outside, thanks to gravity pulling down the corners of my mouth.

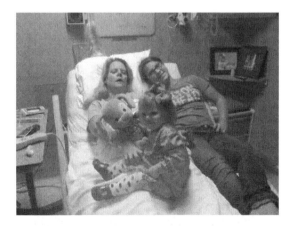

My girls were snuggling in bed with me on the rehabilitation floor. They were my biggest inspiration to push myself to walk again! I loved their visits, and my internal smile was huge in this picture even though I couldn't show it externally.

Chapter 16

Eating and Toileting – the Road to Self Sufficiency

My feeding tube was removed. I was brought my first meal. I will always remember how it looked, smelled, and tasted. It looked like pig slop, but I was told it was pureed beans and rice. It smelled good. The back of the bed was raised, so I could rest my back on it, with a tray in front of me, while I ate. I tried to feed myself with the spoon, but my hand was shaky, my face was paralyzed, and it proved to be messy, frustrating, and time consuming.

Greg took over and fed me. It tasted good. I still had a slight metallic taste in my mouth, but not nearly as strong as before. This time, the taste of the food overpowered the taste of the nerve damage. I ate several small bites, and that was a big milestone. Those bites gave me enough energy to get through physical therapy.

PT in the beginning consisted of sitting upright in a wheelchair, being wheeled down the hall to the gym, being lifted out of the chair and laid on the mats, and having my legs moved and stretched for me. Afterwards, I was wheeled back to my room and encouraged to remain in my wheelchair for as long as I could tolerate before being placed back into a comfortable, flat recline in my bed. I pushed myself to sit up as long as I could. Greg's Caring Bridge entry that Saturday said, *"Wenesday sat in the wheelchair for TWO hours! Yeah! The PT worked her so hard that hopefully she will sleep well tonight."*

My large catheter bag that had sat on the floor was changed for a smaller "sporty" one that wrapped around my leg, and was able to be hidden under my baggy sweatpants. After several days of the sporty catheter, I had an ultrasound. It showed that I was able to completely empty my bladder, and the sporty catheter was removed. When I had to go to the bathroom, I called the nurse's station, and was lifted by a team of two or three techs onto a potty chair in my room.

About a week later, one of my favorite nurses appeared by my bed, and the young nurse with the long, blonde hair was with her. They asked if I would mind if the experienced nurse taught the young nurse how to remove a central line. The young nurse had never removed one before and was eager to try mine. For the first time during my hospital stay, I declined a request for someone to be able to learn. They very readily and politely accepted my decision, and the experienced nurse pulled the central line out of my heart through the tiny holes in my neck while the young blonde watched enthusiastically. My neck was stitched and bandaged, and I was told I would be able to experience a real shower once the wound healed.

Throughout my hospital stay, I missed my dogs and thought about how therapeutic it would have been to have been able to pet them. One day, I told my occupational therapist about missing my furry babies, and she whispered, "You could have Greg drive them to the roof, and I could wheel you to the rooftop to see them." I laughed, "That's a great thought, but they'd jump out of the car and run off to explore. They're huge and spoiled rotten. They'd either get hit by another car or run into the hospital and lick everyone. While they are gentle, they are giants, and they would probably scare a lot of patients."

Greg rescued Kona when Greg and I were dating. A man who worked at Greg's plant in New Orleans found a puppy running down the middle of a busy street. He picked him up and brought him to work on his way to taking him to the animal shelter. Greg saw the puppy and immediately agreed to adopt him. Greg called me, "I just got a puppy! He's adorable! Can I bring him to your house to meet Kayla?" That was the first time Greg and Kayla met. Kona introduced them.

Cindy picked me. My good friends in Louisiana, Michelle and John, had a dog named Stella, who I loved and babysat for when Michelle and John went out of town. When Stella had puppies, her human parents told me I could have the pick of the litter. About a dozen pairs of adorable eyes looked at me, and then one puppy ran toward me with full speed and jumped on my legs. I knew instantly she was the one. Kayla named her Cinderella Ariel, and we called her Cindy.

Greg's boss at work, Jay, had an adult child with special needs who lived with him. Jay had always seemed friendly, but very business-like to me. Jay's soft side appeared in my hospital room. I think it may have been because he was a father who had spent a lot of time with his son in the hospital that he knew the perfect gift to bring me. He brought me a life size stuffed animal dog. It was the size of a body pillow.

As I'd been missing my dogs, the stuffed dog warmed my heart. Jay asked me what I was going to name my new stuffed dog. I looked down at my t-shirt I was wearing that my mom had gotten me. It said "OPTIMISM" on it. I smiled (internally) and answered, "Opti."

I slept with Opti every night for the duration of my hospital stay. Once I returned home, my girls confiscated him from me, and I was glad to relinquish him then. Greg's Caring Bridge entry continued, *The highlight of her day, other than seeing her family, was receiving a huge stuffed dog that she has named Opti (short for optimism). Wenesday has the motivation and determination to get home quickly and fully recover from this horrific syndrome.*

While I was practicing sitting up in between therapy sessions throughout the day, I stared at myself in the mirror. It was nice being able to see myself at will for the first time, but it was also very depressing. My face had absolutely no movement. I smiled at myself, I frowned at myself, and I raised my eyebrows at myself. All my reflection showed me though was a woman with unkempt hair with zero movement in her face and the corners of her mouth pointed ever so slightly downward because of gravity.

Even when I smiled hugely, my reflection looked miserable. The corners of mouth didn't move. I wasn't able to show my teeth at all. My cheeks had no definition. My eyebrows didn't budge. The good news was that any traces of a wrinkle I may have had previously were gone.

That was optimistic me, always looking for the silver lining.

I stared at myself a lot and I tried really hard to make my face work. I wanted to be able to smile at my kids more than anything in the world. It was hard, but I tried to stay positive.

I practiced writing in my notebook, which I still have. On one page, in my messy scribble, I wrote, *"Today is Monday, 11/8/10. I am in the hospital, but sitting up in wheelchair, which is a positive thing."* I made a point to celebrate the baby steps. It was clear that big steps would not be made through leaps, but through countless baby steps.

Chapter 17

Vertical

Being able to sit in a wheelchair, while uncomfortable, was a welcome reprieve from lying motionless. Imagine getting into your most comfortable position in bed (my caretakers were more than happy to arrange my legs and back in any position I requested). Now, stay like that. Don't move an inch. Don't move your legs, your back, your toes, or even flinch. How long is that comfortable?

I had no idea how much I moved throughout the night while sleeping – even tiny movements – until I couldn't do it any longer. I didn't want to be a bother with my call button, but there would always come a time – more frequently than I liked – when I couldn't stand it any longer and I would succumb and push the button. All I wanted was for someone to move my leg just an inch. That tiny movement made a huge difference in comfort.

That had been one of my ongoing struggles since first becoming paralyzed. Sitting in a wheelchair meant that my body was in a novel position and I was actually able to put my hands under my thighs and move my legs a fraction of an inch, which was something.

There were some problems paralysis caused though, that not even sitting up could cure. I had been told from the very beginning about foot drop. Foot drop could result from not standing; it is when the foot falls forward and is no longer able to flex upward. Once it happened, it was usually permanent. As a preventive measure, both of my feet had been placed in hard, blue boots from my very first day in the NICU. The boots had tiny kickstands on them and kept my toes facing the ceiling while I was lying down. They were on my feet around the clock. They had never bothered me until I was in the rehabilitation unit. As more sensation returned, I started to feel the discomfort of my pink skin against the hard, blue boots. Socks were put on my feet under the boots.

Dr. Payne took my boots off, and as I lay in the bed, we both stared down at my feet. They were sitting in an odd position. They were both turned slightly inward. Normally, my feet turn slightly outward to the sides. One of my feet was slightly pointing straight, toward the wall, and not up toward the ceiling. The doctor noted that I really needed to get into a standing position because weight bearing would be the quickest, most effective means of correcting the problem.

The next day, in the therapy gym, Gerardo wheeled me to a standing frame and strapped a harness around my legs and waist. The harness hoisted me up, and my arms rested on the frame, helping the harness support my weight. For some reason, having my legs in a standing position resulted in awful pain and more tears. I wanted to stand. I really, really, really, desperately wanted to stand. It REALLY hurt just to be placed in a standing position even when the frame supported my weight.

At the same time as the pain, as soon as I was stood upright, the entire room started to spin. Gerardo put a blood pressure cuff on me and immediately sat me down.

Crazy spikes in blood pressure are common occurrences with GBS. Mine had become so low, the nurse was immediately called. Blood pressure medicine was soon added to the other drugs I was taking.

I was also given a wide band to wear around my torso and pressure hose to wear on my legs. I remembered joking with my friend Gina who, shortly after turning forty, had to wear support hose after having varicose vein surgery. I'd given her a pretty hard time. Now, I was thirty eight wearing support hose. That was perfect karma. I actually laughed out loud and had to share the story with my caregivers, eager to share it with Gina as soon as I could.

I agreed to try the torture stand (what the professionals called the standing frame) again the next day. It really did look like something out of a medieval torture contraption book. It hurt. Gerardo helped me breathe and count through the pain, much like if I were having a baby. All this contraption did was hoist me up with a harness, so that I was in a standing position, with my legs straight up and down. It supported my weight for me, and Gerardo held on to me for balance. It sounds simple and easy. My body disagreed.

Gerardo then suggested we try something new. He showed me a treadmill with a harness and suggested that the movement of my legs might actually feel better than them just hanging straight. Naturally, I was eager to try it. Gerardo and his tech strapped me into the harness that hugged me very, very tightly around my legs and waist, somewhat like a diaper made out of straps.

When first placed in that position, my back would begin to tilt backward, like I was going to fall. The tech would support my back, and I was able to grab on to a handle in front of me to hold for support and to help keep me vertical. Gerardo would put his hands on my waist and legs. He started the treadmill moving and he moved my feet and up and down in a walking motion. While this too hurt, it was actually less painful than the torture stand.

The treadmill was also fun. While I was only passive in the process, my limbs were moving as if they were functioning. I tried to lift my feet with each stride, and couldn't, but it was ok because Gerardo did it for me. I was so very excited.

I arranged for Greg and my mom and dad to be able to watch me "walk" on the treadmill the next day. I was very proud. This was a huge stride in the right direction. Greg, my parents, the therapists, and even other patients in the gym cheered for me.

A couple years later, my mom confided in me that when she saw me "walk" on the treadmill for the first time, it actually scared her. She could see that I had zero awareness of my body and I didn't know when I was falling over and when the tech put me back upright. She could see that I was not moving my legs or torso at all on my own volition. I was oblivious though, and I was happy to be making progress, no matter how slow. I even asked to be photographed for the first time since I entered the hospital. It was passive, but I was walking!

After a couple days of "walking" in my real tennis shoes, the foot drop worries resolved, and I was able to take long breaks of not wearing the boots while in bed. During a visit from Kayla and Sarah Grace, Sarah Grace actually snuggled up next to me and napped in my bed. That was Heaven! Kayla polished my toe nails for me. I looked down at my pink nails and smiled a huge smile. I know Kayla saw it, even though my face couldn't show it to her. That was really sweet and thoughtful.

I felt much loved by both of my girls. Greg kept making balloons out of surgical gloves and making me laugh. My dad commented how strange it was to hear me laugh, knowing I was genuinely laughing, but to see my face was not moving a millimeter. My sister-in-law, Robin, visited from Louisiana. She somehow knew that sitting in a wheelchair looking up at people all day took a toll on the body, and she gave me a wonderful, unsolicited neck and shoulder rub. The little things are actually the big things. I knew there would be a long road ahead, but was comforted by a returning sense of normalcy.

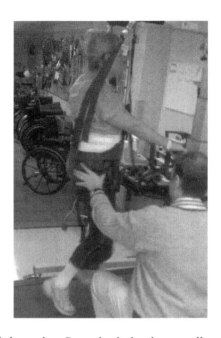

My physical therapist, Gerardo, helped me walk on a treadmill while a harness held me upright. It was scary and very painful, but it felt really good to progress in the direction of being able to walk again.

Chapter 18

The Great Outdoors

My friend and neighbor, Shannon, visited when it was sunny outside, and I told her how I longed to feel the fresh air. At that point, I'd been in the hospital for about two and a half or three weeks. She asked my nurse if she could take me outside, and the answer was yes, as long as we stayed close to the main hospital building and weren't gone too long.

Shannon put a light jacket on me and pushed me out of the door, down the hall, and to the elevator. I was so excited about going on my first field trip! When we exited the hospital door and the fresh air hit my skin, it was amazingly wonderful! I love being outside, and that excursion was really good medicine for me.

The sun seemed unusually, almost painfully bright. Then, I realized I'd been inside with only fluorescent lighting for weeks, and my eyes hadn't been closing completely when I slept or blinked, so it made sense. We added sunglasses to the list of items I wanted brought to the hospital from home.

Shannon wheeled me to an open area on the hospital grounds, and we parked under a red-leafed tree. She sat on a park bench and I sat in my wheelchair. We talked, we listened to the wind blow through the trees, and we watched birds fly and tiny bugs crawl around on the ground. Those are all things I had always taken for granted, but at that moment were very prominent and important.

The next time my family visited, my dad brought me a pair of bright red sunglasses, Kayla pushed my wheelchair, and Sarah Grace rode on my lap. Kayla wheeled Sarah Grace and me through a labyrinth maze that was painted on the ground. Then, Sarah Grace (fifteen months old) hopped off my lap and ran through the maze. I LOVED being outside with my family and friends! I was like a giddy teenager, looking forward to each visit, not only to see the visitor (which, of course, was still the most important thing), but now also to be able to go outside!

Greg wrote about these events on our Caring Bridge site. *"I don't know how we can ever demonstrate our gratitude to all our friends and family for the love, encouragement, prayers, and support. Wenesday continues to make good progress in her recovery, working hard in OT & PT. She has been in the wheelchair each day and it is less painful each time. She continues to eat (semi) solid food and her appetite is growing. Her speech is improving daily and the metallic taste she has had in her mouth the last few weeks is subsiding. She is beginning to taste food again. She has even been outside the last two days soaking up some Vitamin D. Sarah Grace took her afternoon nap in Wenesday's arms, sleeping for hours in the bed with Wenesday, possibly the best therapy yet.*

As all of you know, Wenesday always has a smile on her face. But because the GBS had reached her facial area, she has been unable to smile, even when she is happy and smiling on the inside. She desperately wants to smile again and sooner rather than later. We are praying that her smile returns to her face quickly. Please continue to visit – Wenesday loves to see people. Wenesday tried to type a journal entry, but was unable to do so. I am sure she will have an entry posted soon, so stay tuned. I still read every guestbook entry to her, so keep them coming! We love you, Wenesday! Keep up the great attitude and hard work!"

Another entry from Greg, around the same time, said, *"We have had wonderful help through all of this, but one person in particular deserves special recognition. Kayla has been a wonderful help with her little sister and around the house. She has matured beyond her age the last few weeks and handled this circumstance very well. Thank you, KK!"*

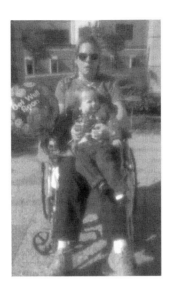

I was smiling really big in this picture even though my face couldn't show it. I was happy to have my baby in my lap, the strength to sit in a wheelchair, my oldest daughter caring for me by pushing my chair, and simply the blessing to be outside after having been indoors for so long.

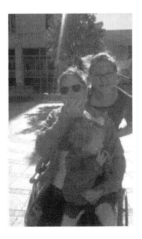

My face wouldn't smile on its own, so my fingers gave it a little boost. I wanted my external smile to reflect my internal smile. I love the ray of sunshine showering us from behind.

Chapter 19

Unrecognizable

The first movements that returned to my legs were knee twitches. Then, I was able to bend my knees a couple inches up, off the bed, toward the ceiling. My upper body was getting stronger too (which we worked on in OT), and I was actually able to grab onto the bed railing and pull my body from one side to the other, making life much more comfortable.

I took a few steps on the parallel bars in the gym, assisted by Gerardo, who held onto me with a belt around my waist, and his tech, who stayed right behind me with my wheelchair. Progress was the best motivator, and I pushed myself hard.

The next day, I took twenty five steps on the parallel bars and also walked on the treadmill! It felt GREAT! Again, the entire gym – patients and therapists - was cheering me on.

It was grueling work – I had never imagined that simply taking assisted steps would feel to my body as if I'd just run a marathon. But, I knew I had to work hard to get better, so I did. I put on a brave face for everyone and tried not to let them know just how much of a struggle it was to try to learn to walk again.

I actually felt really bad that I couldn't smile at my fellow patients in the gym. That was one of the worst parts of it for me – possibly worse than the physical pain. Most of the patients on the rehabilitation floor were older. Some had had strokes, some had broken hips.

There was one young man, probably in his thirties, who appeared in the gym one day. A spot on his head had been shaved, and he seemed to have communication difficulties. I knew that whatever he had been through was probably worse than what I was going through. I wanted to smile at him, but I physically couldn't.

There was a ninty year old woman who was the most popular patient in the gym. She'd had a leg amputated and was learning to get around with only one. She was always upbeat, smiling big, and said, "Hi!" to everyone. She was always dressed like she was ready to go out to dinner – in nice pants and a blouse, wearing jewelry. I apologized to her for not being able to smile at her. She said it was ok and that she hoped I get better soon. I made a point to keep her attitude with me, wanting to be upbeat like her when I reach her age.

After a very hard work out in the gym, Gerardo's assistant wheeled me back to my room. He was a young guy – probably twenty years old – and I could see that he looked up to Gerardo. He was eager to help with anything he could. When asked to get a piece of equipment, he walked quickly, with purpose. When asked to push the wheelchair behind me, he made sure I knew he was right there and that I was safe, helping me to overcome my fear of falling. He always wore fun scrubs with basketball print.

One day, we talked the whole way down the hall as he wheeled me to my room. We talked about our families, and I showed him pictures of mine when we got to my room. I first showed him pictures of my kids individually, and then I showed him a picture of my whole family together. He'd met my husband and recognized Greg in the picture. He pointed to me though and asked, "Who's she?" It was a picture that had been taken only months earlier.

"That's me. That's what I look like in real life." He was very nice and tried to hide the stunned look that uncontrollably popped on his face. Then he said, "Can I ask you a personal question?" I answered, "Of course! I'm an open book!" Then he asked, "What happened to your face?"

My heart broke in two at that moment, but he didn't intend to break it. He didn't even know it had happened. I was sure he meant no ill will at all. He was simply inquisitive. I would have been too.

I calmly explained, "My face is paralyzed from GBS, just as my legs were paralyzed. I have a beautiful smile, with visible teeth; I just can't show my smile now. I can't move my face at all." He asked, "Will your face return to the way it was before?" I answered solemnly, "Nobody I've met has seen bilateral facial paralysis before, and the doctors really don't know, but are optimistic. I REALLY hope my face returns to normal."

He was a good guy. I stayed strong for him because I knew it would hurt him if he were to know that his innocent words hurt me. He left my room with me sitting in my chair in between my bed and the large mirror on the wall.

I stared at my face in the mirror. He was right; I didn't look at all like myself. I looked like a crazed, grumpy woman. I smiled at myself internally; but externally, I looked like a mad woman.

Greg walked into my room, knowing I would have just finished physical therapy. As soon as I saw him, my strong façade disappeared, and I broke down crying. "He didn't even recognize me!" Greg gave me a tight hug first, in order to calm my hysterical crying, and then asked me to explain what I was talking about. He listened, we talked, and I felt better. Greg, as always, was my best source of support and comfort.

Chapter 20

Stretching the Limits

I pushed myself as hard as I could, always trying to do more than what was asked of me. I wanted desperately to get better and to be strong enough to return home to my kids, walking and able to care for them. My back hurt and the nurse gave me a heating pad. My blood pressure was still erratic and I was still getting dizzy every time I first became vertical. I was exhausted, both physically and emotionally, and my physical therapist recognized it.

Greg wrote in Caring Bridge, *"I am sure it is no surprise to anyone that Wenesday continues to improve. There are days that we see more improvement than others, but still always some good news to share. Yesterday, Wenesday walked TWENTY FIVE steps! She also spent some time on the treadmill. Her rehab today was a little less strenuous, as she may have worked a little too hard the previous few days. Wenesday had to be reminded that the tortoise wins the race, and that this is a marathon and not a sprint. But, as you can probably imagine, Wenesday's spirit, motivation, and determination to recover may occasionally drive her too far too quickly."*

In the gym, Gerardo taught me how to transfer myself from my wheelchair to my bed with assistance. First, I learned using a sliding board. The first time I was to put it into practice, I was in my room with three techs helping me. It was hard to imagine being able to scoot myself across a tiny board to the bed a couple inches higher than the chair, even with assistance.

Fear gripped me. I was going to fall. I was going to break bones. I was going to be in the hospital even longer.

These techs were my favorites. They regularly got me dressed and put me on the toilet. They cleaned me and helped feed me daily. We had talked about my life and their lives. One of them had let me counsel her on an issue she was having with a friend. She gifted me with the good feeling that comes from helping another person, even while I was feeling pretty helpless myself. I completely trusted these three ladies.

Still, I was panicking. I begged for them to just lift me onto the bed like they normally did, but they said the therapist instructed them to make me use the transfer board. I wanted to comply, I wanted to learn, I wanted to progress, but I was terrified. I started to hyperventilate from crying so hard.

My favorite tech, a woman probably in her fifties, got down on my level and told me to look at her in the eyes. She told me they could wait all day, but we weren't going to do anything until I stopped crying and composed myself.

I started taking deep breaths and calming down. I knew the three of them genuinely liked me and wanted to help. They looked at each other, then back at me, and in unison said, "We're like Allstate. You're in good hands!" It was a cute play on the insurance company's tagline, and I knew they meant it. I was too upset to laugh, but I appreciated their lightening the mood, and I trusted them.

I listened to their instructions and placed my hands on the board, slowly raising myself from the chair while they held onto a belt around my waist and assisted in lifting my body. One of my feet got stuck behind a foot pedal on the chair though and didn't move with the rest of my body. They assisted, and I made it safely onto the bed. From there, I grabbed onto the handrail, scooted toward the middle of the bed, and slowly lay down. They lifted my legs onto the bed, and turned me in the right direction.

I had successfully transferred myself. Even though the room was spinning from my change in orientation, the accomplishment felt good. I used the board, with assistance, several times after that when I needed to move from the bed to the wheelchair and back. I was always a little apprehensive about it.

As my strength improved drastically over the coming days, thanks to intensive physical and occupational therapy, Gerardo taught me a new trick. It was called a standing pivot transfer. It was technically more difficult and physically demanding, but I liked it much better. I wasn't relying on a board that I was afraid might pop out from underneath me.

Gerardo held onto my torso with his hands and braced my knees with his own as I pushed myself up with my arms. I stood for just a few seconds, shuffled my feet (a new accomplishment!) around a few inches toward the bed, and with his help, gently lowered myself. Success! I moved myself from the chair to the bed, and while I definitely needed assistance, this time nobody had to actually lift me up. I felt very accomplished. If I had to return home in a wheelchair, this would be the type of transfer I'd want to use at home.

Once the wound in my neck closed, I was cleared to take a shower. First, it was with my occupational therapist. Later, it was with a tech, so that I could work on strengthening my upper body and my fine motor movements during OT. I was so excited about the thought of a real shower! It seemed like forever since I'd had one, and it was one of those things that I knew would feel great and make me feel more like myself; it was also one of things that in my pre-GBS life, I had taken for granted.

The shower chair looked funny. It was a wheelchair with a large hole in the middle of it to allow the water to drain. I had been getting used to sitting up in a wheelchair, but this one proved to be a little trickier. The chair seemed very hard and uncomfortable, and sitting in it the first several times caused pain. It was well worth it though.

I was wheeled down the hall and into the shower. The warm water poured down on me, and it was Heavenly. It was almost enough to cause me to forget the pain in my back and behind from the unyielding chair. I washed my face and my other reachable parts with a washcloth, and my hair and the rest of me was washed for me. I had long ago gotten over any qualms with modesty. It felt really good to get a real shower.

My friend and hairdresser, Heather (a different Heather than my friend who was a former physical therapist), visited me for the first time the day she knew I was getting a shower and getting my hair washed. She appeared with brushes, combs, scissors, and a bag of assorted chocolate. My hair was pretty long then, half-way down my back, and had become a frizzy, matted mess. I asked Heather to cut it all off for me. She refused – and for that, I am thankful – but, she did give me a trim and straighten my hair while I sat in the wheelchair. I looked in the mirror and a brand new person, with pretty, shiny hair, looked back at me. As I smiled, my reflection still frowned, but it was a much prettier reflection – one much more closely resembling the real me than the one I had been seeing.

That was also the day a Greek restaurant first opened its doors in our small town. I had often said to my friends that one of the biggest things I missed about living in a larger town was Greek food. Holly surprised me by delivering a vegetarian meal from that restaurant to my room while I was in my physical therapy session. It was waiting for me when I returned to my room with a happy note taped to it. I also had a hospital lunch delivered. Heather stayed and ate with me - she had the hospital salad and I had some delicious bite sized spanakopita (Greek spinach pie). I later found out that Heather had refused to accept a penny from Greg for driving to the hospital to trim and style my hair.

When my friend, Julie, had moved from Tennessee to Texas a year earlier, I missed her and I missed her famous sour cream sugar cookies. Julie mailed a huge batch of them to me. They were delicious! I had enough to eat and enough to share. I was able to share with both my visitors and caretakers. One of my favorite nurses confided that nurses weren't supposed to eat treats from patients, but I talked her into it. The look on her face when she tasted the moist, sweet cookie, feeling like she was sneaking something, was priceless! Julie had gifted me with the ability to treat the people who had taken such good care of me, and that made me happy!

Greg arranged for my mom to stay at our house on a weekend night, and he and I had a slumber party. He came with my laptop that played DVDs, an assortment of my favorite movies, and some European chocolate. We shared the hospital bed and snuggled as much as my limited movement and discomfort would allow, held hands, and watched "My Big Fat Greek Wedding." I only had room in my stomach for a few bites of the dark chocolate, which is very unusual for me, but it sure tasted good. He slept on the sofa in my room. Having a date night with my husband was just what the doctor ordered. It felt right. I felt special and loved. It was fun waking up with Greg in my room.

I had been quite depressed, and it seemed like Greg, my girls, my parents, and my friends had been conspiring to make me feel better. It was working. Life in the hospital was a roller coaster ride with some really good days and some really low days. Visitors were always highs for me.

Therapy was strenuous and stressful, but also a little fun because I got to push my limits in creative ways and see gains, even though they were often tiny. Returning to my empty room and staring in the mirror, trying to smile at myself, but with my face not budging, was always a big downer. Each time, I'd fully expect to see some movement in my mouth, cheeks, or forehead. After all, my legs were moving more and more – even slow progress was definite progress. My face showed no progress at all. Each time, I was surprised and disappointed. Surely, after the success I'd had walking a certain number of steps in therapy, and with as happy as I felt about that, I'd be able to smile. But, I couldn't.

Speech therapy (ST) was added to my PT and OT. My speech therapist was a very compassionate woman named Lydia who told me she'd seen me in the gym, had heard about me, and had wanted the opportunity to try to help me. She, like all of the others, had not seen bilateral facial paralysis resulting from GBS before. She had, however, worked with many stroke patients before who had facial paralysis.

My speech was still a little slurred, but my voice was almost back to normal in strength. Lydia admitted I was a challenging case. What would help my speech would be to learn to move my mouth in certain positions. The catch, of course, was that my mouth didn't move into those positions.

She showed me what she wanted me to practice – big, exaggerated smiles, frowns, kissy faces, eyebrow raises, etc. My face didn't budge. She said that even though I couldn't see any movement, I should continue practicing those things in the mirror. She didn't want to see my nerves regenerate, but my face still not work properly due to muscle atrophy. She believed that practicing the movements, even though my face wouldn't do them, was good exercise. I did it several times a day, every day.

Lydia put ice on my face and rubbed my skin vigorously. She researched and tried new therapies with me each session. Nothing seemed to be working, but she was tenacious, and I think she wanted to see my face move almost as much as I did.

Gerardo went above and beyond the normal call of duty for me. With permission from my doctor, at the end of my physical therapy sessions, he would stay late, it seemed cutting into his lunch time, and work with me on my face.

Gerardo's job as a PT was to get me walking. That's what we worked on during my normal PT hours. He also made it his job as a good person and my new friend to try to get me smiling. Many times, during PT, I'd lie on the mat and cry. He'd ask if the leg raises or whichever exercises I was doing were that painful. I'd confide in him that most times, I was actually crying because I had caught a glimpse of my face in the mirrored ceiling. I'd been smiling, thrilled at my leg lift accomplishments, but my reflection frowned back at me.

I think Gerardo understood how important my smile was to me. He began electrical stimulation on my face. He explained that he would use an electric current to try to stimulate my muscles into contracting. He used a device that looked like a small TENS unit. He allowed a current to run from the unit, through his body, and into mine. His finger touched various points on my face. He shocked precise spots - the corners of my mouth, my chin, my cheeks, the outer corners of my eyes, and my forehead. We both watched intently. We were both disappointed when my face didn't budge. We weren't giving up easily though. We continued this novel therapy throughout the rest of my hospital stay.

A neuropsychiatrist interviewed me and determined that I was officially moderately depressed. People usually label me as happy, laid back, and upbeat. Depressed was a new label for me. I didn't like it. It was depressing.

The process was eye-opening too. I told the neuropsychiatrist that in my life before getting to be a full-time mom, I had been a rehabilitation counselor for eleven years. I had a master's degree, a state license, and a national certification to help people with disabilities. I had never dreamed that I'd be the patient on a rehabilitation floor at such a young age.

I thought about one of my clients who I'd treated with a "tough love" approach years earlier, who'd told me he wished one day I had a disability. As my tears streamed when talking about my new disabilities, the neuropsychiatrist asked me what I would tell a patient in my shoes if I were her rehabilitation counselor. If I were my counselor, what would I tell myself? All I could come up with was, "It's ok to be sad. It's ok to cry." He asked what else I might say. I answered, "Don't be embarrassed about crying. It's ok. It makes sense that you're sad right now." He looked hopeful, "Wouldn't you tell your patient that things WILL get better?" Oh, yeah, good point. I hadn't even thought about that.

The fact that such a simple truth had not even popped into my head confirmed for me that I really was in a low place. I should have known the answer he wanted me to give. I should have been more upbeat. I really was depressed.

He asked if I thought there were other people in the hospital at that moment in worse positions than me. That, I could truthfully answer in a fairly positive way right away. "Of course there are. I can see people being transported in the helicopter through my window. I would bet they're in really bad shape, since they need air transport. The worst thing I can imagine are the parents who are surely somewhere in the hospital with their really sick children. My children, thank God, are healthy."

I thought of one of my therapists. When Amy, my regular OT, got married and went on her honeymoon, another one of the OTs worked with me. One day, during my session, she asked why I was crying. I told her that I missed my children. Stephanie would take them to the hospital to see me later that day, but I wanted to be home with them. My therapist was able to empathize all too well. She missed her children too. She confided in me that she had lost a son to a car accident. Her other son took the loss of his brother very hard, and as an indirect result, my OT later lost her only other son to drugs. My children were healthy and safe, and for that, I was very, very, very thankful.

It was November, and Thanksgiving was fast approaching. I practiced writing in my notebook. I really wanted to write a list of things I was thankful for, but I had writer's block regarding that upbeat idea. I wrote first, in my shaky handwriting, with tears streaming, a list of what I wanted other people to be thankful for, things I had lost and didn't want other people to take for granted....

- *Your ability to smile.*
- *Even your ability to frown; it means you have expression.*
- *Your ability to walk and run and skip.*
- *Your ability to toss and turn when you can't sleep at night; it means you can move.*
- *Your ability to hold your children in your arms safely.*
- *Your ability to breathe and your heart to beat regularly.*
- *Your ability to go outside at will.*
- *Your ability to feel the fresh air on your skin.*
- *Your messy house; it means you are LIVING in your own home.*
- *Your ability to talk and write, to communicate.*
- *Your ability to go to the potty on your own.*
- *Enjoy your everyday abilities and appreciate them...they could be gone at any time.*

Once I completed that list, I was able to write a list of things for which I was thankful at that moment....

- *My family!*
- *I have the best husband, daughters, bonus son, mom, dad, sister-in-law, honorary sister, and doggies in the world.*
- *My catheter being removed.*
- *My ability to eat and taste food.*
- *My friends.*

- *Prayers from my family, friends, and even friends of friends.*
- *Every day baby steps.*
- *Twenty five steps!* (I wrote this list after proudly taking a record twenty five steps).
- *Clean hair.*
- *Flowers, cards, and balloons.*
- *The ability to roll onto my side.*

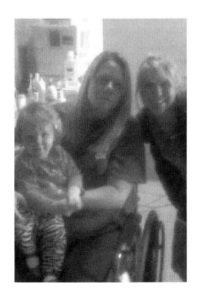

The nurses had been braiding my hair to keep it from getting matted. My friend and hairdresser, Heather, came to the hospital and trimmed and straightened my freshly washed hair. It felt so good to look a little more like myself. I was smiling big in this picture, even though it's not visible on my face.

132

Chapter 21

Big Strides

When Amy returned from her island wedding, I was excited for her and asked her to bring her wedding pictures. After our OT session, she told me about getting married barefoot on the beach and showed me her photos. I started crying again. I realized that the chances of Greg and me going to St. Thomas for our five year anniversary with all of the people who'd gone to our wedding were greatly diminished. Our fifth anniversary was in only a couple months. I didn't know if I'd even be able to walk by then. I was happy for Amy and mad at myself for making everything about me – that wasn't like me – that was the depressed me. That realization gave me more motivation to get better and I pushed myself even harder.

In OT, I learned to use a tool with a long handle to take off and put on my socks and shoes. I used machines to strengthen my arms. I completed puzzles, putting nails into holes, to work on my dexterity and speed. Eventually, I stood against a table and completed a puzzle, working on balance.

In PT, I worked on leg stretching and strengthening. We worked on walking and balance. One day, when Gerardo was out, another PT filled in. We watched another woman in the gym walk for the first time with a walker. He suggested, "Wenesday, let's try you on a walker!" I was shocked and excited. Until that point, I had been practicing on the treadmill and the parallel bars. "Are you serious?" He nodded enthusiastically. "Ok! I want to try!"

The PT held the belt around my waist, the tech pushed the wheelchair behind me, and I slowly shuffled forward, leaning on a walker, lifting it and setting it back down with each tiny step. I was walking! I was really walking! It was a GOOD day!

Greg's Caring Bridge said, *"Wenesday has been in the hospital for 23 days. Looking back, it is remarkable to realize and to comprehend all that Wenesday has endured in such a short period. She went from typical stomach flu-like symptoms to numbness in extremities, pain, almost total paralysis, ICU, feeding tubes, and total dependence on others for the basic needs that we all take for granted. This weekend, Wenesday continued her journey back; she is eating (and enjoying) some of her favorite things like chocolate, she can sit up on her own, and she walked about 16 feet using a walker! Yeah! She is making progress daily, although she doesn't always see the progress. We thank our Father in Heaven for all the changes we witness daily even if they don't SEEM significant at that time. We know that all the little changes fit together to make one BIG change! Please continue to pray first and foremost that her facial paralysis is only temporary and that her awesome smile returns to her face quickly. Those that know Wenesday know how important this is to her."*

The next day, I couldn't wait to share with Gerardo my accomplishment. He was visibly happy for and proud of me. He was eager to try the walker with me, and I was eager to show off my new skill. This time, I walked and walked and walked with the walker. Gerardo asked if I was ready to stop, but I was on a roll, "No, I want to keep going!" He ecstatically responded, "Ok, let's keep going! Tell me when you're ready to sit!"

My legs felt numb, tingly, and painful from my toes to just above my knees. The more I walked, the more intense the tingling. I asked Gerardo if that was ok, and he reassured me, "It's good. Your nerves are waking up. It won't hurt you." So, I kept going. As I walked past the nurse's station, everyone looked shocked, smiled, and cheered me on. They all clapped for me.

I walked so well with the standard walker that I got to trade it in for the sporty model only a day later – a walker with wheels! It felt AWESOME! I knew I was making big strides! I was proud.

Greg's Caring Bridge entry documented, *"The progress never ceases! Some days, Wenesday's progress is as big as Kilimanjaro; other days, we are searching relentlessly in the haystack for her progress. Today, she climbed the mountain! Wenesday walked 145 feet with her walker! The whole length of the hospital hallway! Yeah! Everyone on the rehab floor has been more than impressed with her progress. In the rehab gym, Wenesday is the "life of the party." Imagine that! She will try to have "fun" with everything she does and her recovery is no exception! We continue to be thankful for all the prayers and support from our family and friends."*

One of the "fun" things Greg was referencing was when I sang the Filipino anthem. I was in the gym, working on leg strength, talking to Gerardo (who was originally from South America), Mark (whose family was originally from The Philippines), and Mark's patient about my childhood in the Philippines. I told of how every morning at my school on base, we had to sing both the American and the Filipino anthems. I sang what I remembered of the Filipino anthem in Tagalog, the language of the Philippines. Everyone in the gym seemed to be listening, and even though I couldn't smile, the only child in me secretly enjoyed being a ham. Mark said, "Wow! I've never heard a white person sing that!" His reaction made me laugh.

I had also reached a point in my progress where I was finally able to have fun in therapy. I was no longer worried about backsliding or reinjuring myself, my pain had dropped to a bearable level, and progress was finally measured in large enough to be noticed increments. It truly was fun to practice my new skills. It was fun to be vertical. It was fun to walk. And I was proud of all that I had accomplished. It wasn't easy, and I was doing it!

The next logical step was, of course, learning to walk without a walker. Gerardo held tightly to the belt around my waist, the physical therapy assistant with the basketball scrubs walked behind me with the wheelchair, and I walked!

I looked like a toddler taking her first steps. I was shaky and wobbly at first, but got steadier with each step. Balance was no longer something that just happened automatically – I had to concentrate and move my body slightly in one way or another to make sure I stayed upright. It felt like I was learning to ride a bike without training wheels. Again, as I walked past the nurse's station, mouths dropped. Therapists and patients in the gym clapped their hands. I felt like a rock star! I was walking on my own!

The next game (exercise in disguise) I got to play involved Gerardo walking next to me, holding my belt, while I played ball with the man in the basketball scrubs. We threw and bounced a ball to each other while I walked. I wobbled at first, and quickly became proficient. I was able to walk, balance, throw, and catch a ball! I joked that the only thing I couldn't do simultaneously was chew gum. I was all smiles…on the inside! I felt like I had just run my first marathon!

In the gym, Gerardo practiced falling down and getting up with me. He told me that once I went home, I would likely fall down a time or two, and he wanted to be sure I was able to get myself up off the floor. I was able to use furniture as an aid to help me pull or push myself up.

We also practiced walking on stairs. I held the railing on one side and Gerardo's hand on the other. I was to use my strongest leg first going up, and my weakest leg first going down. The mnemonic device Gerardo taught me to help me remember was, "the good leg goes up to Heaven and the bad leg goes down to Hell." I told Gerardo I wanted to be able to walk up and down the stairs while carrying Sarah Grace. He assured me that we would practice carrying weights eventually.

I was allowed to keep my walker in my room. That meant I was able to walk to the bathroom without calling for assistance. That was a huge and important milestone.

Greg's Caring Bridge summed up the latest and greatest events, *"I apologize for not updating the last couple of days. The fact is if I updated every time Wenesday made progress, then I would be updating throughout the day, every day! Wenesday has been making miraculous strides in her recovery. On Thursday, she walked 1,000 feet with the walker! YEAH! But wait, THAT wasn't enough, so she decided to tackle walking up and down the stairs! Wow! But don't stop reading this yet. On Friday, Wenesday walked WITHOUT a walker! Woohoo! Oh, did I mention that she did it WHILE BOUNCING A BALL??!! Wenesday is the "talk of the rehab floor." They had to reset her goals because she is by far exceeding THEIR plan. I guess they didn't realize who they were dealing with! And, Wenesday is now considered "independent" in her room. Her recovery is truly miraculous and we must honor our Father in Heaven for His hand in our lives."*

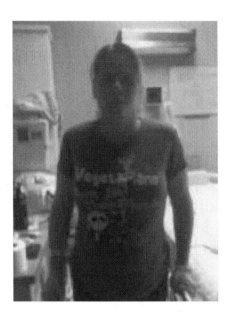

In this picture, I was standing with a walker in my room for the first time! What a glorious achievement! My internal smile was huge! And, I was wearing my "vegetarians don't eat their friends" t-shirt that my daughters gave me.

Chapter 22

Thanksgiving

My family typically celebrates Thanksgiving twice annually. The Sunday before is when we have the big feast. Our extended family comes to our home. Everyone gets to choose at least one dish. The choice factor means that along with the traditional turkey, we also have vegetarian options and unique items. One year, Kayla chose a peanut butter sauce on broccoli that she'd seen in a cookbook. It turned out to be delicious and became a staple at our Thanksgiving meals for a time. On Thanksgiving Thursday, we usually go to my parents' house and have a very tasty and extravagant, but much smaller meal.

The Sunday before Thanksgiving, my mom picked up everyone's special orders from my favorite restaurant and brought it to the hospital. We had too large of a group to eat in my room – Greg, Kayla, Sarah Grace, my parents, and Greg's mom who was visiting from California – so my family wheeled me down to the hospital dining room. Sarah Grace rode in my lap, which she thought was quite an adventure! My mom had even brought a tablecloth and fancy napkins, which made it feel festive. I had eggplant parmesan and a grilled romaine salad with blue cheese dressing. Everyone talked and laughed and lingered. It almost felt like a real Thanksgiving. It felt incredible to know that I was loved enough for everyone to do that for me.

After the meal, I had to go to the bathroom. I had only ever done that in my hospital room. Rather than wheeling through hallways and elevators, my dad suggested I try to use the bathroom in the dining room. It sounds like a little thing, but it was a big deal. My mom helped. There were bars in the handicapped stall, and I was successful in transferring from the wheelchair to the potty in the public restroom. It felt like a huge victory and a big step towards being able to go home sooner. It was a great day!

The thought of spending Thanksgiving Thursday, and then my thirty ninth birthday a week later, in the hospital was starting to become bearable. I realized I wouldn't be alone and it would be ok and even fun. I didn't have to do it though. On Monday, I was told that I was being sprung from the hospital on Wednesday, the day before Thanksgiving! Of course, everyone had fun playing with the wording that Wenesday would go home on Wednesday. It seemed appropriate.

I awoke early Wednesday morning, full of excitement about going home, gratitude for the fantastic care I had received, and pride for all that I had accomplished. After signing some paperwork, while waiting for Greg to pick me up, I stared all around my room, wanting to remember it. Every wall was covered in cards, banners, artwork...outpourings of love that meant the world to me.

I used my walker to get to the walls and I began the process of peeling things off the walls myself. I knew Greg planned to do it, but the independence felt good. I was careful not to tear anything. Greg came with boxes and smiles. I said good bye to and hugged my favorite caretakers who were on duty. My favorite tech shouted, "I love you!" as I zoomed away on my walker. Greg helped me into the car and loaded my stuff into it. I couldn't wait to get home! It was a sunny, gloriously beautiful day!

It felt surreal stepping inside of my house. It felt like I had been gone for a very long time. I was greeted with hugs from both of my girls and my mom. I felt like I had won the lottery! Greg held my hand walking through the foyer, and then I was able to hold onto furniture and walls for support, and not have to rely on my walker in my house. I still couldn't carry Sarah Grace. I was thankful that Stephanie had agreed to stay and help, and drive me to outpatient physical and speech therapy, while I continued to recover.

That night, Greg held onto my left hand while I held the railing with my right hand, and I walked upstairs to Sarah Grace's room. I was able to sit in her plush chair and rock her to sleep for the first time in over a month. I looked down at her with a huge smile. She returned the smile at the exact right moment! I don't know how she saw past my perfectly still face, but she did. She knew I smiled at her, and she smiled back. That was a perfect moment! Once she dozed off, Greg and Kayla took her from me and put her in her crib.

I was still my girls' mom. They were my babies and we had a bond that no paralysis could break. Of course, Kayla understood about my face, but I had been really worried about Sarah Grace. She saw my smile. She knew it was there, even when it wasn't visible to the eye.

Everything was going to be ok. I got to sleep in my warm bed that night with Greg next to me. I was home.

On Thursday, instead of us travelling to Memphis, everyone came to my house. We had A LOT to be Thankful for that Thanksgiving! That evening, I took over Greg's job and typed a Caring Bridge entry by myself:

"I AM HOME!!!!! I love this Caring Bridge site, and I have LOVED hearing all of your entries, which Greg read to me daily in the hospital. They kept me optimistic and energized and hopeful and connected. THANK YOU all for posting on here! THANK YOU, Tara, for setting this up! Thank you, Greg, for being you! Your updates on this site were so well written, and your caring for and loving me unconditionally was/is beyond anything I could have ever dreamed. You are truly my knight in shining armor! Thank you, Kayla, for stepping up to the plate and being so loving and helpful! Thank you, Sarah Grace, for giggling with me even when I can't smile back at you yet! Thank you, Mom and Dad, for EVERYTHING!

There are so many people I want to thank! I spent 33 days in the hospital. I endured more physical pain and more fear during that time than I ever had in my entire life. I want to thank God for helping me through this ordeal! Of course, without Him, I wouldn't have gotten through it. I don't want to just echo Greg's earlier post, but I truly want to thank everyone who prayed for me and my family, everyone who visited me in the hospital, brought food to my family, sent me cards, sent flowers, brought balloons, offered my hubby and/or daughters hugs, sent me homemade cookies all the way from Texas, surprised me with Greek food after physical therapy, offered words of encouragement when I was down, shared their similar past experiences with me, held my hand when I was scared, drove Kayla to school, helped us find the nanny from Heaven, trimmed and styled my hair in the hospital.... The outpouring of support my family and I have received has warmed my heart and touched me in ways I can't even begin to explain. I can't begin to thank everyone enough. That having been said, I must also thank my doctors (my neurologist, cardiologist, pulmonologist, hospitalist, and rehabilitation doctor), physical therapists, occupational therapists, speech therapist, techs, nurses, CNAs...all wonderful, compassionate, knowledgeable, and great at what they do!

I have come a long way in a little over a month. I have come from a 10 day stay in the neurological ICU, paralyzed in my legs and face and weak in my arms and hands, with a feeding tube and central line, with the probability of having to go on a ventilator and pacemaker, to now walking on my own and holding my children in my arms in my own home, taking a shower on my own, and eating anything I want (while I do enjoy having lost over twenty pounds on the feeding tube diet, I wouldn't recommend it). Still, I have challenges to face. My walking isn't yet perfect and I can't yet put Sarah Grace into or take her out of her crib; my face still isn't working the way it should, and I still can't smile. Most of you know that I love to smile, and it hurts me to just look at people with a blank face. If I may ask, please do continue to pray for my family and me...prayers have worked so far, and I believe they will continue to do so!

Again, thank you all! Some of you I see regularly and some of you I haven't seen in years. All of you, I appreciate and love! Thank you, thank you, thank you!"

Chapter 23

Life at Home

Of course, I was overwhelmingly grateful to be home, but I was also on an emotional roller coaster. When it was time to go to sleep at night, I was very happy to be at home with my family, but I was also filled with anxiety. I still saw and heard the beeping machines from the neuro ICU when my eyes closed. It felt like the hospital was real and home was an illusion. Soon, the dream morphed into feeling more like reality, and I was at home being at home. I resumed my normal life, but with much more appreciation for it.

I attended outpatient physical therapy and speech therapy three times a week for about six weeks. There, I practiced walking without a walker, and eventually climbing stairs while carrying a lopsided weight that was made to resemble a baby, weighing the same as Sarah Grace. I made tremendous progress. Greg and I did physical therapy homework. At first, we practiced walking outside with him holding me with a belt for balance and stability, and we too practiced climbing stairs. Later, we practiced independent walking with Greg staying close for safety.

The outpatient speech therapist was friendly and enthusiastic. He acknowledged that he had never before treated bilateral facial paralysis using an electrical stimulation (e-stim) machine. He said that he had wanted to try it on himself before hooking me up, so he had done it at home the night before we met.

This machine was a little different from what Gerardo had used in the hospital. This machine had round pads which were placed on specific spots on the face and attached to wires. The therapist had turned the machine to an intensity of three (ten was the maximum) and said he had felt pain, and his face had contorted into odd and exaggerated expressions. We started with the machine on a level three on me, and gradually turned it up to a ten, but I didn't feel it, and my face remained motionless. It was disheartening.

After several sessions, the outpatient speech therapist determined I could shock my face at home just as easily as he could do it at the clinic, so I was sent home with an electrical stimulation machine and instructions. I used it for several additional weeks, but the lack of noticeable progress was incredibly frustrating and depressing, so I discontinued it.

I was willing to try anything that could help my smile. I heard about a Chinese acupuncture doctor in Jackson, so I made an appointment. I told myself that acupuncture has been around for thousands of years, so while it's not common in the United States, there must be something to it. I went in with an open mind.

Without hesitation, the acupuncture doctor said he felt confident he could help both my paralyzed face and my tingly toes. His office staff promptly took my payment, and then he put needles in my face and on my feet, attached them to a machine, and sent electricity into my body. I didn't experience any miracle relief, and I bled where the needles were placed. The vision of acupuncture I had in my head didn't include blood. I returned one more time, and then stopped going, not believing it helped me at all.

One day, as I was looking at the milk in the grocery store, a lady with beautiful red hair approached me, smiling. "You probably don't remember me, but we met briefly at a moms' group at church a while ago. My name's Kati." She went on to tell me that her husband, Stephen, was a chiropractor. They'd heard my story and had prayed for me. I asked, "Can he help my face?" She answered, "I don't know, but I'm sure he would love to try."

The first thing Dr. Stephen Wilks said to me when I walked into his office was, "I prayed for you this morning." That made the fact that he was about to twist and pop my neck feel a little less scary. He said, "I've honestly never treated anyone for facial paralysis, but I did some research, and I think chiropractic care could help." The chiropractic manipulation was helpful. I saw some gradual improvements in my smile while I was under Dr. Wilks' care, and I know my neck and back benefitted too.

While it wasn't the instant miracle cure for my smile I'd hoped for, it did help. The most important blessing to me from the entire experience though was an unexpected one. Stephen and Kati had a daughter Sarah Grace's age, and our families became close friends. Their daughter, Wesley Kate, ended up being Sarah Grace's first best friend.

My face took a lot longer to show improvement than the rest of me, but it did improve. Gravity held both corners of my mouth slightly downward, making me look like I was sad or angry. There was no movement at all in my forehead, cheeks, or around my eyes. The first sign of improvement was tiny, but it was something. The left corner of my mouth moved up ever so slightly when I smiled. It wasn't enough to make it look like a smile, but it was enough to make a difference. When I smiled, my mouth became horizontal on the left and continued to sag downward some on the right. That was the first of many baby steps for my face, and I was happy about it - any improvement, no matter how slight – was better than nothing.

Stephanie, our nanny from Heaven, had agreed to continue helping us after my return home. She seemed to intuitively know what to do to help. She allowed me to take care of Sarah Grace as much as I could, and she was right there the second I needed help or to rest. I was able to be a mom and also be a recovering patient simultaneously. She treated me with the utmost respect, and even when it was probably obvious I needed help, she waited for me to ask, which I appreciated. That way, I felt like I had some control over my life and my taking care of my youngest daughter. She drove Kayla home from school and to her activities. She drove me to and from therapy and took care of Sarah Grace while I was in therapy. Stephanie and I had a lot of time to talk, and we became close. She had quickly become a member of our family.

I had lost about twenty pounds, and a group of friends had all pitched in and given me a generous gift card to a department store to buy some clothes that fit.

Stephanie, Sarah Grace, and I headed out for our field trip. I had scored a handicapped parking tag when released from the hospital, and Stephanie pulled into the last handicapped spot on one aisle. There were more spots on the next aisle. A woman pulled up behind us with a handicapped license plate. She saw Stephanie, with her young, healthy body and blonde hair, and made a lot of wrong assumptions. I don't think she even noticed that Stephanie was driving me. The woman stuck her head out of her vehicle window and yelled at Stephanie, "You're parking in a handicapped spot! You're handicapped in your head!"

Stephanie is one of the sweetest, most caring people I've ever met. She would never take a handicapped spot if not for a legitimate reason. She was shocked and asked me if she should give up the spot, drop me off at the door, and park somewhere else. I told her to stay put; I had as much right to that spot as the other woman did. That lady whipped her car into a spot on the next aisle, equally close to the door. We watched as she got out and walked with a cane to the door, faster than I could go.

When we saw her in the store, it occurred to me that I had the power to make her feel bad. Part of me wanted to say, "You yelled at my nanny who was driving me that she is handicapped in her head. As you can see, I am handicapped in my face. I would smile at you right now, being a friendly person, but I physically can't. You really hurt my feelings when you yelled that at us – were you saying I'm handicapped in the head?"

She looked unhappy, and it was evident that she was either having a bad day or was simply a miserable person. Even though her walking was faster and easier looking than mine, I was instantaneously aware that my life was more blessed than hers. I felt sorry for her. Rather than trying to make her feel bad, I decided to give her a little grace. I smiled at her, but she couldn't tell. She gave me a grumpy look and continued shopping. That was one of those moments when it was clear that an internal smile is much more important than an external smile. I needed that reminder.

My lack of ability to smile affected me more than my lack of physical agility. Stephanie, my girls, and I took pictures with Santa at the mall one day as Christmas approached. The photographer kept telling me to smile. We all said, "We are smiling!" and she finally snapped the picture. I didn't want to explain myself to a mall Santa photographer, but I also felt bad knowing she probably thought I was a grumpy mom, not smiling.

On that same day, I bought Greg a shirt from a rather pricey men's store. The sales clerk seemed genuinely concerned about me and asked me numerous times if everything was ok. I did explain to him that I had been paralyzed recently and that my face was still paralyzed. He seemed to understand. I felt better knowing he knew I wasn't unhappy, even though I looked it; in fact, I was in the Christmas spirit and very happy shopping for gifts. When I checked out though, he said, "Maybe Christmas will bring you enough joy to allow your smile to return." He meant well, but he just didn't understand. I wasn't not smiling because I wasn't happy – I was happy – I was not smiling because my face would not physically move in that way. I wanted to wear a sign around my neck that said, "I AM smiling on the inside!"

Life's timing is sometimes unbelievable. Stephanie's boyfriend, Mike Slater, moved to California because of an amazing career opportunity to host a radio show in San Diego shortly after I was released from the hospital. I was able to listen while Stephanie cried. She was thrilled for Mike, but was going to miss him terribly. It was actually a blessing to me to be able to be in the helping role for a change.

After I completed physical therapy, had adjusted to my new normal, was able to care for myself and my children, and was able to drive again, Stephanie made the decision to move to California. She had taken a break from school shortly before we first needed her. She decided to move over a thousand miles away shortly after we stopped needing her. Her window of availability was perfect. The timing confirmed that Stephanie truly was a gift to my family from God. There was no other explanation.

A few years afterwards, we were invited to Stephanie's wedding. It was her day; she was the bride; and yet, she went out of her way to make us feel special. As she and her brand new husband walked out of the church, she spotted my family and me in the crowd for the first time and was visibly excited to see us. We felt loved at that moment. Then, during her reception, she took Sarah Grace by the hand and walked her to the dance floor. There, Stephanie, Mike (the groom), and all of the groomsmen – there were a lot of them – danced an entire song with my sweet little Sarah Grace while Kayla, Greg, the rest of the wedding guests, and I watched and smiled. Stephanie made Sarah Grace feel like a princess. Stephanie is a beautiful person on the inside and the outside and I am so happy to know that she has found her knight in shining armor!

About five months after GBS, my girls and I visited Tara and her family in Charlotte, North Carolina, where we spent a day at the National White Water Center. While Tara and her boys played with Sarah Grace, Kayla and I jumped into a raft to ride the waves. White water rafting was a lot of fun until suddenly, our boat capsized.

I was bobbing up and down in my life jacket, being swept downstream, with waves constantly splashing my face. I didn't see Kayla. Where was Kayla? For just a split second, I panicked. I immediately realized my legs weren't yet strong enough to fight the current, even though I'd been a very strong swimmer during my life. I spotted and grabbed our overturned raft. Within a minute, our guide was holding me in his capable arm. "Where's my daughter? I don't' see her!" I gurgled, with some water in my mouth and waves continuing to wash over my head. He pointed to the shore.

She'd been one of the first people rescued with a rope and was high and dry. Relief! Some other guides helped right our raft. Back in the boat, I explained to my rescuer that I had been paralyzed only a few months earlier, and that my legs were still weaker than normal. I guess I should have told him that from the beginning, when during the safety briefing he'd asked if anyone had any disabilities, but I hadn't. I'd thought I was strong enough for it to not be relevant. I was wrong. I was still happy though. Suddenly being tossed into massive waves and a strong current was certainly an adrenaline rush! Kayla held me steady as my jelly legs wobbled on the shore at the conclusion of our ride. I was a little weak, but revved up! I told Kayla the only thing left to do was to dry our hair in the wind – via a zip line!

We checked in with Tara, Sarah Grace, and Tara's kids, and we drank some water and ate a quick snack for energy replenishment. We then headed to the zip line area. It was quite a climb up a rope spider web to the top of the zip line tower. Kayla zoomed to the top and waited for me. My climb was much slower, but steady, and I made it to the top! It looked higher from the top than it did from the ground. My heart started to race. I told myself my new mantra, "I learned to walk again! I can do anything now!"

I smiled (outwardly, the best I could) at Kayla, and stepped off the ledge. In my memory, I screamed excitedly, "Whooooo hoooo!" In Kayla's version of events, I screamed in terror, "Aaaagggghhh!" Either way, when my feet hit the ground, it was an amazing feeling of accomplishment! Once again, I'd pushed my body and my fears, and surpassed the previous limits. I felt great! I gave Kayla, Sarah Grace, Tara, and Tara's kids all proud high fives!

We visited family and friends in Louisiana. Jennifer's daughter, Erin, was six years old at that time. Her mom and dad had prepared her for what to expect when she saw me, but no words could prepare a child for the drastic change she would see in my outward appearance. Erin was polite and sweet all through breakfast. Afterwards, she sat right next to me on a bench outside and put her hand on my arm. She looked into my eyes with a big smile and the enthusiasm of a cheerleader. The pure heart of a child spoke, "Come on, Ms. Wenesday, try to smile! I know you can do it! Just try really hard!"

Over time, my smile improved very gradually. It's hard to see improvement when staring in the mirror every day looking for it. It takes a lot more time and requires a lot more patience than waiting for water to boil. I learned to look at my teeth as an objective measurement. My original smile showed all of my pearly whites.

After GBS, I couldn't initially show any teeth when I smiled. One day, the bottom of my top left middle tooth was barely noticeable. That was a good day. Months later, another tooth was visible on the left side. My facial improvement has not been over hours or days, but over months and years. At the time I am writing this (three and a half years post GBS), when I smile, four of my top left teeth and two of my top right teeth are visible. The medical literature suggests that with GBS, most noticeable gains are seen within the first two years. My smile is objective proof that improvement does continue past that window.

My toes have remained numb and tingly, and I can only bend one toe on each foot downward. That hasn't stopped me from being physically active. I exercise, walk, run, and climb. My balance may be a little off, but I was never very graceful, even before GBS.

Prior to my paralysis, getting pedicures was an adventure. The bottoms of my feet were so ticklish that I would have to use my hands to hold my legs down and stop my reflexes from jerking my legs away. After GBS, I was able to get pedicures and just stay still. I hadn't really thought about that until one day, a few years post GBS, my leg jerked from ticklishness and I had to hold it still with my hands. I loved it! Even the feeling in my toes and my reflexes are still gradually continuing to improve.

I haven't let GBS keep me down. To the contrary, I have made a point to appreciate all of the abilities I have. I have walked, run, skipped, hiked, biked, zip lined, swum, gone white water rafting, played tennis, and even taken hardcore Cross Fit classes since recovering. When we walk around the neighborhood and Sarah Grace gets tired, I am able to carry her on my back now. I don't take any of those things for granted.

Kayla has never been embarrassed of my face around her teenage friends, something I'd initially worried about. Greg has never been embarrassed to take me to work functions and walk with me on his arm since my smile changed, something I had worried about. Sarah Grace has never seemed to notice that my smile is different, and it hasn't changed her smile, something I had worried about.

Life has gone on and has blossomed. Whether or not my hair is perfect when we leave the house in the morning isn't important. Whether or not I've told Greg good morning, played with Sarah Grace, and paid attention to Kayla before I leave the house is important. I knew that before, but it's much clearer now. How I think my external smile looks is far less important than how I know my internal smile is doing.

Most days are super good days. I know I am blessed beyond measure. That is where my thoughts dwell ninety eight of the time.

I do have moments though of sadness and reminders. My family and I went to Disney World three years after GBS. Disney World is a magical place, and we had a magical time. Sarah Grace was young enough to believe that all of the princesses were real. Kayla had fun figuring out where the cameras were located on rides and planning funny photo bombs. One of my favorite pictures is from our last ride on our last vacation night. Kayla and Sarah Grace sat in the front seat on Splash Mountain, with their eyes and mouths open wide in delight, while Greg and I closed our eyes, arm in arm, tilted our heads to the side, and pretended to be asleep in the seat behind them. That vacation was a dream come true and my GBS had not even entered my mind until one specific morning.

As we entered Magic Kingdom, the fingerprint reader didn't recognize my print, so I was told to smile for a security camera. I gave a big smile, not thinking twice about it. The cast member was a friendly guy and in a kidding manner said, "That's a weird smile!" My heart broke. I know he wasn't trying to be mean. He probably thought I was being silly, making a silly face, and he was trying to be silly with me.

It was the reminder though that I didn't need that my smile didn't look genuine on the outside, even when it was huge on the inside. During the rest of the trip, I was a little self-conscious, constantly wondering if the friendly princesses who went out of their way to make us happy knew that I really was smiling. Still, we had an awesome time – one of our best vacations ever - and I made a conscious effort to not dwell on that one moment.

When we returned home, I did send an email to Disney customer service just so that such an incident wouldn't happen to anyone else. While facial paralysis is rare, I know people who have had strokes or other neurological events go to Disney, and I wanted the cast members to be sensitive to them. The response I received was immediate and positive. A supervisor called me, sincerely apologized, and promised the cast members would be trained on the issue. I felt good about that.

Chapter 24

Should I explain?

To this day, I struggle with whether or not to address the elephant in the room. I don't want to immediately turn a conversation to me, but if I meet a new person, I tend to spend a lot of time worried about whether or not they perceive me to be friendly. I have learned that I really don't have to explain myself to the people I meet briefly, like a server at a restaurant, or the UPS driver delivering a package to my door. At first, it mattered to me, but then I realized that usually those people are in such a rush completing their jobs, they don't usually take the time to notice the expression on my face anyway. When I meet a new friend or when I interview for a job (paid or volunteer), the question of whether or not to tell becomes very important.

Shortly after I returned home from the hospital, I jumped at the opportunity to serve in our local soup kitchen through the Jackson Service League. It seemed like the perfect opportunity to give back to the world that had given so much to me. The soup kitchen is expertly run by a hard working pastor the community affectionately calls Father Dan. My scheduled shift was the first time I met Father Dan. At that time, I didn't want to draw attention to myself, and I thought if I didn't address my smile (or lack thereof), my personality would kick in, and people would magically know that my face was paralyzed and that I was smiling on the inside. Such was not the case.

Father Dan briefed the volunteers on their duties and prayed with the group before the lunch hour. He then talked for a few minutes that seemed like an eternity about the importance of a smile. "The food is great, but what people really come here for is the warmth of our volunteers. It is very important that each of you smile at our each of our customers; yours may very well be the only smiles they see all day." It was clear that he was concerned about the look on my face, the corners of my mouth that drooped slightly downward. After the second such well-meaning pep talk, with my heart heavy, my friend Christy explained for me to Father Dan about my smile. A lightbulb visibly went off in his head and he understood for the first time. He walked over to me, hugged me, explained that he hadn't understood, and said a quick prayer for me. From that moment, I knew it was a good idea to address the elephant.

Even as my smile progressed, there were similar incidents. When I returned to graduate school to become a teacher, the professor in my first class addressed our small class, "it is important to make your students feel welcomed and loved. Some people don't like to smile, and that's ok." I knew that even though my voice and actions were enthusiastic and warm, she was confused about what she saw on my face. After that class, I talked to her privately and explained about my face. From that moment on, I felt like she liked me more. She understood and accepted me. I asked her if she thought I should address my face from day one to students and teachers when I taught school. She asked, "Would it make you more comfortable?" I answered, "I think it would. That way, people would know why I wasn't outwardly smiling and they would understand that I am warm and that I do care about them." She responded, "Then, I think you should address it from the beginning."

I have made many new friends in the four years since my GBS. At least two of them have acknowledged, now that we know each other well, that when they first met me, they wondered if I genuinely liked them because of the only partial smile on my face. I know now that addressing the elephant in the room makes a lot more sense than trying to ignore it.

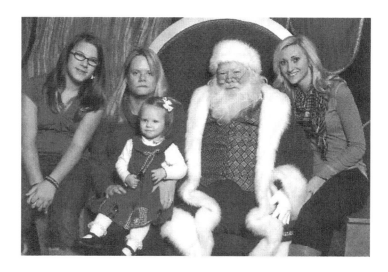

This picture was taken a couple weeks after I returned home from the hospital. My internal smile was huge. I was with my daughters, our fabulous nanny, and Santa Clause! Of course, externally, I looked less than enthusiastic. The Santa photographer kept telling "us" to smile. Even though the photographer couldn't tell, my smile was progressing by this point. The right side of my face remained motionless, but if you look closely, you can see the left corner of my mouth was showing a little movement.

Chapter 25

Helping Others, Thanking Those who Helped Me, and
Celebrating Milestones

About a year after my initiation into the scary world
of GBS, I was able to visit a newly diagnosed woman
named Sara in the hospital. Sara was a friend of a friend.
When I first met her, she'd had a tracheotomy and was on a
ventilator. While she was unable to speak, it was clear that
she was happy to see me. I told her I'd been paralyzed too,
and then I said, "Look what I can do now!" I jumped up
and down.

I know I brought her comfort, but perhaps no good
deed is truly altruistic; the joy the visit brought me, being
able to help another person in that position, was unexpected
and immeasurable. I visited her a second time, while she
was on the rehabilitation floor. I asked, "Has anyone taken
you outside yet?" She responded, "No! Can we do that?"
We secured permission from her nurse, and I, with my head
held high, pushed Sara in her wheelchair on her first field
trip to the great outdoors!

I was also able to see many of my previous
caregivers during those visits and hug and thank them.
David, the NICU nurse who'd made me stay in the torture
chair hugged me and volunteered, "I may have seemed
mean at the time, but I only pushed you for your own
good." Mark, who had done my initial physical therapy
evaluation, didn't immediately recognize me. I put my

hands to my face and pulled my expression down with my fingers to resemble the face he knew. He instantly recognized me then, and exclaimed with a smile, "Wenesday!" It felt good to know that my face had changed so much in the right direction that I'd become unrecognizable!

A couple years after that, I was able to visit a newly diagnosed man named Ronald in his fifties. He was numb and tingly, but able to move his legs. I watched him walk on his walker and joked with him, nudging him to stand with no hands. He did, and he smiled. That visit felt good too.

I began visiting people in the hospital with GBS from early on in my journey, to provide them with hope. Of course, I've continued, armed with more information and tools, since having become an official liaison. One of the most memorable people I've met in that process is a girl named Elexys.

Elexys was only 10 years old when she was hospitalized with GBS and pancreatitis. When I first met her, she was dependent on a ventilator for breathing, in a lot of pain, and very scared. I brought her a small pink stuffed animal named Opti Junior and told her the story of my Opti. I jumped up and down at the side of her bed, and explained that only a few years ago, I had been paralyzed like her.

After some time, I got to witness her taking some of her first steps in the hallway with her physical therapist. She pushed back tears and trudged forward, slowly, but purposefully. She endured more than any child should ever have to, and she did it with grace. I cried tears of empathy for her in my car before and after each visit, and smiled big for encouragement when I was with her. I believe I was able to provide her and her grandmother comfort, information, hope, and realistic expectations. I know she provided me with many blessings. My stepson once said there is no true altruism; that people benefit when they help others. I think now that he is probably right, and that is ok.

As of this writing, I have had the opportunity to visit seven different people newly hospitalized with GBS. I felt sad for all of the people I got to meet in the hospital. Knowing what they were going through, I had cried for them in the parking lot before getting out of my car. I wiped my tears, touched up my make up, and put on my game face. By the time I made it to their rooms, I was strong, smiling, energetic and enthusiastic. By the time I left them, I felt genuinely happy to have been able to be of some comfort and hope to them. Helping others truly is the best therapy.

I spent the first anniversary of my GBS diagnosis and hospitalization in Gatlinburg, TN with Betsy, one of my best friends and old college roommate. It was coincidence that our vacation fell on my GBS anniversary date, but it felt like fate. It was the most beautiful time of year to visit the Smoky Mountains. The trees were covered in orange, yellow, and red leaves.

Betsy and I live in different states and see each other only once every several years, but it felt like we had never been apart. Talking came easily, and we had a lot to catch each other up on, so we didn't stop talking during the entire weekend. One year to the day of my paralysis, Betsy and I hiked to the top of Laurel Falls. Then, we climbed the rocks to the bottom of the roaring waterfall. When my balance got shaky, Betsy offered a helping hand. I stood on a rock at the base of the fall and looked up at how far I had come.

I felt like I was in the clouds! I hiked 2.6 mountainous miles and traversed boulders on the first anniversary of my paralysis. I felt capable of accomplishing anything. What an awesome feeling! I was filled with gratitude and pride, and so very happy to be alive, healthy, and active.

About a year and a half after my hospitalization, a Guillain-Barré Foundation International chapter hosted a Walk and Roll fundraiser in Charlotte, NC. My best friend since childhood happens to live there. Greg, Kayla, Sarah Grace, and I were able to visit and stay with Tara and her family. We all participated in the walk together. I loved being there with my family and my honorary family (Tara is like my sister; she is Kayla's Godmother, and her son is my Godson). Walkers/runners were given gray shirts, but walkers/runners who were GBS survivors were given bright red shirts. We survivors were able to spot each other easily.

I met a woman who'd had GBS while pregnant. I met kids who'd had GBS. I met people who were still paralyzed and using wheelchairs (hence the "roll" in "walk and roll") due to GBS. Most dear to me, I met a man from

North Carolina and a woman from Holland who each had facial paralysis from GBS, like me.

GBS occurs in about one of every one hundred thousand people. Bilateral facial paralysis from GBS occurs in about one of every million people. I had met GBS survivors before – they'd visited me, and I later visited them – in the hospital. That walk in Charlotte was the first time I'd met other people with facial paralysis from GBS. While I was sad for them, and would never wish it for them, I was also selfishly happy to finally meet others walking in my shoes.

It was immediately clear that the three of us understood each other. We all had the same anxieties and insecurities. I often wondered when I met new people if I should tell them about my face, so they wouldn't think I was giving them rude looks, or if I should just ignore the elephant in the room, so they wouldn't think I was wanting to become the center of attention with my story. It turned out they both also struggled with that same dilemma. What I was going through was perfectly normal in my situation. We hugged and took a picture together. Our smiles were very similar. I was no longer the only one in the world. It was comforting and strangely uplifting.

My second anniversary was spent at home alone, staring in the mirror at my crooked smile, pouting. I wanted to do something more productive, but couldn't peel myself away from the mirror. I tried in earnest to form a big, toothy smile, but nothing worked. My face was forever changed. I cried a lot that day. I gave myself permission to mourn the loss of my original smile again, but I also vowed to always mark that anniversary with something special, and to not succumb to self-pity in the future.

By the time my third anniversary rolled around, I had developed a passion for playing tennis. Three years after my paralysis, I was crowned "queen of the court." I joked about it with my tennis friends, but it truly felt amazing to be running around in a tennis skirt, successfully hitting balls over the net on that important date. I was happy. I was healthy, active, and with friends. My husband and daughters smiled with me that night as I enthusiastically recounted my tennis success at the dinner table.

On that date, I wrote a Facebook status: *"Today is my 3rd anniversary of being diagnosed with GBS. Three years and one day ago, I had never even heard of Guillain Barre' Syndrome. Three years ago, I was terrified and in a whole lot of pain. I couldn't sit, stand, walk, or even wiggle my toes. I didn't know if I would ever walk again. My face fell flat and expressionless even though I was experiencing a lot of emotion. Since then, I've cherished every moment with my family and friends. I have the best husband, daughters, bonus son, parents, family, and friends anyone could ever hope for! Since October 23, 2010, I've hiked up a mountain and down a waterfall. Since then, I've gone white water rafting and zip lining. Since then, I've ridden horses. Since then, I've walked in a GBS 5K fundraiser. Since then, I've participated in Cross Fit classes. Today, I'm playing tennis. I've experienced milestone moments with my kids I once wondered if I'd ever live to see. My smile isn't what it used to be on the outside. I'm still a little self-conscious about my face and how the nerve damage has changed my expressions. My smile on the inside though is bigger than it has ever been. I have had and am still living an amazingly wonderful, blessed life, and I am thankful every day. Today marks the 3 year anniversary of my new appreciation for my awesome life. I am happy. When you see my smile not looking very strong on the outside (but much stronger than it appeared 3 years ago!), just KNOW that I AM smiling big on the inside! Happy 3 year anniversary to me! And a huge thank you to all of my family and friends who have prayed for me, offered me a shoulder to cry on, and made me laugh through it all. I love each of you!"*

I began college in 1989 as an education major, but talked myself out of teaching. When my youngest child entered pre-K, my husband suggested it was time for me to return to work after eight years of being a full-time mom. All I could imagine doing was teaching. I love being with, talking with, and teaching children. And I want to still spend summers as a full-time mom.

Even though I have a master's degree from LSU Health Sciences Center, it is in an unrelated field, and a teaching degree required starting from scratch. Three and a half years post GBS, at age forty two, I enrolled in graduate school at the University of Tennessee at Martin. I bought a pretty backpack, learned the school's software programs, refreshed myself on writing in APA style, and so far, I have completed my first two semesters with a 4.0 GPA.

I am very much looking forward to a teaching career! It's never too late to pursue a dream. I plan to live my life to the fullest. I have learned that life is a gift and should be spent doing what makes a person smile.

I spent my fourth anniversary of GBS at one of my favorite places on Earth doing something that I love! I completed the formal training at a conference center at Disney World to become an official GBS-CIDP Foundation International liaison. I also was able to attend the foundation's symposium, which drew experts from around the world. I learned how to help other newly diagnosed people and their family members survive and thrive. I learned how to more effectively educate the medical community, hoping to spawn earlier accurate diagnoses, earlier treatment, and better outcomes.

The song "Circle of Life" from Disney's "Lion King" kept playing in my head. It felt like I had come full circle. Perhaps the reason for having gone through GBS was so that I could bring hope, encouragement, and joy to others. I felt very blessed.

My husband and our good friends, Chris and Alison Weaver, accompanied me to Florida. Of course, the trip wasn't all work; there was a lot of play too. We rode roller coasters, dined at Epcot's Food and Wine Festival, and even wore costumes to Disney's Not-So-Scary Halloween party. I dressed as Cinderella, and Greg dressed as my prince. Alison dressed as Emma Swan, and Chris dressed as Captain Hook from the ABC series "Once Upon a Time."

At the beginning of the training, each new liaison (there were about eighty of us) stood up and briefly stated whether they'd had GBS or CIDP, when, and where they lived. It was sobering. The obvious suddenly registered in my brain seriously for the first time – every person in that room had been affected by GBS or one of its variants.

Some of the liaisons in the room had gotten GBS forty years earlier, some had gotten it that same year, some people were affected when they were very young, some were affected when they were retirees, and one person had GBS while she was pregnant with other young children at home. I was reunited with Patricia, the first woman with facial paralysis like mine who I'd ever met. She's Dutch, has a beautiful accent, and lives in her home country of Holland. I had met her at the GBS walk in Charlotte, NC a few years earlier, and was thrilled to see her again.

The symposium drew five hundred participants from forty nine states and nineteen countries. At lunchtime, I sat at an empty table. Randomly, a woman approached and asked me if the seat next to mine was taken. I invited her to sit, and we began talking. Within a few minutes, she was hugging me. Her name was Susan, and she lived in Greensboro, NC. She too had facial paralysis, and I was the first other person with it who she'd ever met. She hadn't realized it when she first asked me if she could sit at the table.

With five hundred people eating lunch, Susan happened to walk up to me randomly. I couldn't help but believe that God's hand was in that meeting. I introduced her to Patricia. The three of us are members of an exclusive club, and we benefitted from comparing notes. Each of them has struggled, like me, with whether or not to address the elephant in the room. There's comfort in knowing we're not alone.

One of the speakers and participants at our training, Santo Garcia, was an occupational therapist who has CIDP. Chronic Inflammatory Demyelinating Polyneuropathy (CIDP) is, in a nutshell, a chronic form of GBS. Santo was passionate about helping others. He summed up the camaraderie quite well. He said, "Unless you've had to have someone else wipe your butt for you after you've gone to the bathroom, you can't truly understand." I thought he made an excellent point.

A little more than four years after my initial GBS diagnosis, Greg and I had the incredible opportunity to celebrate our ninth wedding anniversary at the awesome Ritz Carlton in Dove Mountain, Arizona. On our first day there, Greg played golf with some of his buddies from work. I decided to go on a short solo hike on the mountain trails surrounding the hotel.

As I climbed up the rugged terrain, over boulders, and next to giant cactus four times my height, I felt an incredible sense of empowerment and accomplishment. As my view of the hotel in the distance got smaller and further away, I couldn't help but be proud of myself. I was climbing a mountain! A rough mountain! By myself! I couldn't help but remember that only four years earlier, I hadn't been able to walk. That realization never gets old. It was exhilarating!

About an hour into the walk, I caught a glimpse of movement out of the corner of my eye and saw what looked like a salamander. I pulled the trail guide that the hotel had given me out of my backpack for the first time in order to try to identify the creature. It was then that I learned that in addition to the cute and small animals, there were also coyotes and four different kinds of venomous snakes in the area.

That might explain why I had walked past a few signs warning people not to hike alone, which of course, I had blissfully ignored. I decided to head back down the mountain with plans to return with Greg. My descent was a little faster than my ascent, since my adrenaline was rushing, but I loved every moment of it. Once again, I had climbed a mountain post GBS. I had the feeling that there wasn't much I couldn't do. When Greg returned with me, he was shocked and worried that I had done that by myself, and impressed and awed that I had done that by myself. I smiled a big smile.

Today, I am left with tingling toes, a changed face, and a deep appreciation for life's blessings. I can walk and run and climb. I can use the bathroom by myself. My external smile is not symmetrical or full, but has progressed to the point that it is obvious when I am smiling or frowning, which is a huge leap in a positive direction. I can raise my eyebrows and a couple laugh lines have returned around my eyes. My eyes still twitch some when I am tired or when I eat, but I am thankful that my eyelids fully close now when I sleep at night. I have learned that if I squeeze my cheeks together with my hands, I am able to whistle again. When I make a kissy face, I feel the muscles in my face strain, but I am able to give and receive kisses.

I treasure the extra time I get to spend with my family. I savor the sounds of my youngest daughter's giggles, treasure the insight my oldest daughter has during our occasional serious conversations, and rejoice over the bond I feel with my bonus son. I am in awe of my children's beauty both inside and out, and I am thankful for my husband.

Kayla was born happy. Not much bothers her. She has empathy for all, and is able to understand other people's perspectives in a way that is beyond her years. There have been many times when, after a long day, she has sat down and announced that she's not going to do anything else productive, but just relax for a little while. Sarah Grace will have an age appropriate melt down, and after a full day with me, not respond to my trying to calm her down. Without being asked, Kayla will swoop in and save the day, despite her own tiredness. She'll sit next to her baby sister, crying hysterically over not getting a third dessert, and calmly ask, "Sarah Grace, can I paint your nails? We can use my new polish that you like." And just like that, Kayla makes our home peaceful again. Not much is black and white in Kayla's eyes; she sees a lot of gray, which adds to her compassion for others. She's extremely smart and excels academically. She has a great sense of humor. She knows all of the words to almost every Disney song. She finds a reason to make people laugh at even the most stressful times. She is a true friend, an amazing role model/sister, and an incredible daughter! I've really enjoyed her teenage years, watching her bloom. She plans to major in speech therapy in college, and I know she'll be a blessing to all of her patients!

Sarah Grace has a love of life that I can't adequately describe. She has a natural ability to read other people's emotions and a genuine desire to help them feel happy. At age five, she wants to become a St. Jude doctor when she grows up so that she can help really sick children. She loves animals too. It's not uncommon for me to have to wait, even when we're in a rush, for her to move ladybugs and June bugs out of the way in the garage so I don't run them over when I back out the car. She is always very careful to include all of her friends on the playground and make sure that nobody feels left out. She is full of love and kindness, and brings joy to all who encounter her. She's uncommonly humble and generous. When I say, "you're so beautiful," she very sincerely counters with, "you're even more beautiful!" She's creative and has an infectious laugh. Even strangers have commented on her gentle spirit. She's also a natural athlete. I have had so much fun watching her push her way past the boys to get to the soccer ball. She is an awesome daughter!

Ryan is compassionate and loving. It is very important to him to always do the right thing. He loves to read and to learn. He enjoys analyzing people and situations. He studies life. He's not content knowing that things are the way they are; he seeks to learn why they are the way they are. He is about to embark on an adventure of a lifetime and move to beautiful, mountainous Colorado with his girlfriend. I hope we'll get to visit him there a lot! He's a great bonus son (our term for beloved stepson).

I am very thankful for all that my husband does for our family, and my love for him has reached depths I couldn't have fathomed before. Greg teaches our family about love and hard work. Greg loves us unconditionally. He works hard to support us financially. He stands up for us. He builds art out of wooden fence boards for us. He can fix anything that breaks in the house. He is the best boo boo kisser, Band Aid applier, and warm snuggler in the world. He's even a fabulous cook who ensures no meat touches my food. He has carried me when I couldn't walk, interviewed Kayla's perspective dates while wearing a shirt that said, "DADD – Dads Against Daughters Dating," taught Sarah Grace to ride a bike without training wheels, and had impromptu guitar jam sessions with Ryan. He even regularly forgives our dogs after they destroy our backyard garden he spends hours planting. He is my perfect life partner, my soul mate.

Kona is our German shepherd/Rottweiler mix, and Cindy (short for Cinderella Ariel) is our yellow Labrador retriever. They've always been giant lap dogs, sweet and gentle. When I came home from the hospital, their love and loyalty shined. Neither of them let me get any further than three feet away from them. They followed me everywhere and snuggled with me the moment I sat down. Their personalities mirror Greg's and mine. Kona has Daddy's yin and Cindy has Mommy's yang. Kona is our protector and alerts us when the UPS truck is a block away or when another dog dares to walk in front of our house.

He would never let anyone hurt his family. Cindy is laid back and goes with the flow, and is always up for a play date. She has soulful, green, human-looking eyes. The two of them are best friends, constantly licking each other's ears, and even lying down with their paws crossed over each other's, as if they're holding hands.

I bask in the warm blessings of my family and friends. I appreciate each step I walk up a swing set and each swing I take with a tennis racket. I am thankful when I am able to throw Sarah Grace in the swimming pool and when I'm able to walk around the neighborhood with Kayla. I take time to notice the perfection of each imperfect petal on a flower outside. I savor the taste of chocolate on my taste buds. Life has become more vibrant since GBS. These feelings of accomplishment and appreciation never get old.

I am excited to see what God has in store for me on my fifth anniversary! I've learned that the future usually holds things even grander than I could ever imagine.

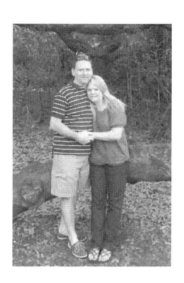

This picture was taken a few months after I got out of the
hospital. I love this picture because it captured my leaning on
Greg and him holding me up. He was my rock during my
illness. Also, my smile had improved quite a lot.

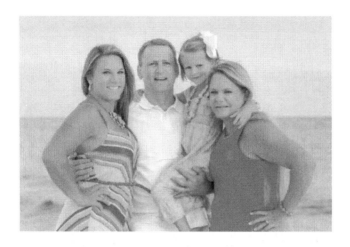

This picture was taken almost four years after getting GBS. My smile continues to improve.

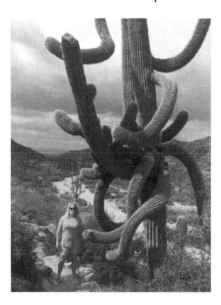

I climbed a mountain of rough terrain and giant cactus by myself!

A Special Request

This is the first book I have ever written and published. I'd love to get it into the hands of as many people as possible in order to increase awareness of GBS. If you loved this book, and if it helped you in any way, please leave a positive review on Amazon's website.

Thank you!

Made in the USA
Columbia, SC
19 October 2020

23064771R00104